Fundamentals of Ethnic Hair

Crystal Aguh • Ginette A. Okoye
Editors

Fundamentals of Ethnic Hair

The Dermatologist's Perspective

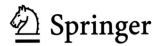

Editors
Crystal Aguh, MD
Assistant Professor
Department of Dermatology
Johns Hopkins University School
of Medicine
Baltimore, MD, USA

Ginette A. Okoye, MD
Assistant Professor
Director, Ethnic Skin Program
Department of Dermatology
Johns Hopkins University School
of Medicine
Baltimore, MD, USA

ISBN 978-3-319-83351-4   ISBN 978-3-319-45695-9   (eBook)
DOI 10.1007/978-3-319-45695-9

Printed on acid-free paper

This Springer imprint is published by Springer Nature
The registered company is Springer International Publishing AG
The registered company address is: Gewerbestrasse 11, 6330 Cham, Switzerland

Foreword

When Drs. Aguh and Okoye first told me of their plans to publish a book about "ethnic hair," I was enthusiastic in my support. There is a real need to educate all physicians about ethnic hair practices so that we can better evaluate and counsel our patients. As a white, male dermatologist from a small town, I can remember my sense of ignorance when I was first confronted with scalp and hair problems in patients of other ethnicities. My self-education was pieced together over many years and is certainly not yet complete.

We need not feel ignorant any longer, because *Fundamentals of Ethnic Hair: The Dermatologist's Perspective* provides "one-stop shopping" for our self-education. The book has many strengths including a very broad scope of topics and extremely helpful images. Although the text is intended for a medically savvy audience, a professional beautician would benefit from exposure to the basic science of ethnic hair care and to the hair loss conditions that their clients might experience. Our patients who wish to self-treat or self-educate might also find this book to be a useful resource. The dermatologist will be gratified to find an explanation of the most distinctive hairstyles as well as the many "this is what it looks like" illustrations. Exhibiting some "cultural awareness" engenders trust in our patients, which translates to improved compliance with treatment.

The authors are to be applauded both for tackling this important subject and also for creating a very readable and "user-friendly" book. Just looking at the illustrations is an education in itself.

Leonard Sperling, MD, Col, MC, USA (Retd.)

Preface

Many of our patients present with complaints of hair breakage or hair loss. This is not unusual, as studies have shown that alopecia (hair loss) is among the top five complaints in patients with ethnic skin. For a majority of these patients, developing a healthy hair care regimen is a critical part of the treatment plan. This requires an intimate understanding of the unique properties of ethnic hair as well as the most common hair care practices among different racial and ethnic groups.

In this book, the reader will learn about the biological differences in hair structure among different races as well as find a detailed discussion about hairstyling practices and their potentially damaging effects on the hair. Additionally, we provide practical management recommendations from a dermatologist's perspective. We believe this book will be helpful not only to dermatologists but also to cosmetologists, hair professionals, and anyone else who has an interest in hair care. We truly hope you enjoy our book.

Baltimore, MD, USA

Crystal Aguh, MD
Ginette A. Okoye, MD

Acknowledgments

The editors would like to thank their husbands, Chike Aguh and Stephen Okoye, for all of their encouragement and guidance during the writing of this book. This would not have been possible without their unwavering support.

We would also like to thank Alessandra Haskin for her contributions to this book which extend far beyond the chapters she coauthored.

Contents

Part IV   Hair and Scalp Disorders Secondary to Hair Care Practices

Part V   Special Cultural Considerations

Contributors

Chika Agi, BS University of Pittsburgh School of Medicine, Pittsburgh, PA, USA

Crystal Aguh, MD Department of Dermatology, Johns Hopkins University School of Medicine, Baltimore, MD, USA

Cynthia O. Anyanwu, MD Department of Dermatology, University of Texas Southwestern Medical Center, Dallas, TX, USA

Katherine Omueti Ayoade, MD, PhD Department of Dermatology, University of Texas Southwestern Medical Center, Dallas, TX, USA

Rawn E. Bosley, MD Doctor's Approach Dermatology & Surgery, Okemos, MI, USA

Kayla St. Claire, BA University of Illinois at Chicago College of Medicine, Chicago, IL, USA

Chelsea Rain St. Claire, BS Michigan State College of Human Medicine, Grand Rapids, MI, USA

Nashay N. Clemetson, MD Department of Dermatology, The Johns Hopkins University School of Medicine, Baltimore, MD, USA

Brandon E. Cohen, BS NYU School of Medicine, NY, New York

Jean-Claire Powe Dillon, BS Department of Dermatology, University of Texas Southwestern Medical Center, Dallas, TX, USA

Nada Elbuluk, MD Ronald O. Perelman Department of Dermatology, New York University, New York, NY, USA

Alessandra Haskin, BA Howard University College of Medicine, Washington, DC, USA

Alice He, BS Johns Hopkins University School of Medicine, Baltimore, MD, USA

Mamta Jhaveri, MD, MS Department of Dermatology, Johns Hopkins University School of Medicine, Baltimore, MD, USA

Ginette A. Okoye, MD Department of Dermatology, Johns Hopkins University School of Medicine, Baltimore, MD, USA

Part I

Structure and Function of Hair

Chemical and Physical Properties of Hair: Comparisons Between Asian, Black, and Caucasian Hair

1

Alice He and Ginette A. Okoye

Introduction

Although the fundamental structure and function of the hair are similar among all races, there are important anatomic and molecular differences that contribute to the unique characteristics of ethnic hair and impact its health and management. Hair researchers have generally classified hair into African, Asian, and Caucasian subgroups [1]. Although this may be an oversimplification, this classification scheme is used in this chapter for the sake of uniformity. These racial subgroups may hold true when discussing the structure of the hair, but when discussing hair management and cosmetic product selection, the relative curliness of the hair may be more important than race.

Hair Structure

The epidermal component of the hair, called the hair shaft, is the portion of the hair that exits the scalp. The dermal components of the hair include the hair follicle (also called hair bulb or hair root) with its stem cells, blood supply, sebaceous (oil) glands, and inner and outer root sheaths (Fig. 1.1a).

A. He, B.S.
Johns Hopkins University School of Medicine, 733 N. Broadway,
Baltimore, MD 21205, USA

G.A. Okoye, M.D., M.D. (✉)
Department of Dermatology, Johns Hopkins University School of Medicine,
5200 Eastern Avenue, Suite 2500, Baltimore, MD 21224, USA

© Springer International Publishing Switzerland 2017
C. Aguh, G.A. Okoye (eds.), *Fundamentals of Ethnic Hair*,
DOI 10.1007/978-3-319-45695-9_1

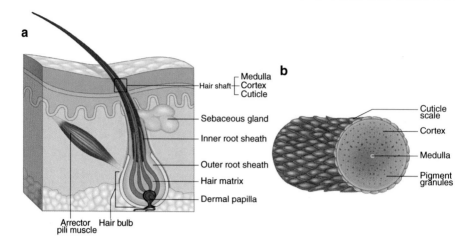

Fig. 1.1 (**a**) Longitudinal section of the hair depicting the epidermal and dermal components. (**b**) Cross-section of a hair shaft depicting the relationship between the three layers of the hair shaft (epidermal component)

Anatomy of the Hair: Cuticle, Cortex, and Medulla

The hair shaft is the part of the hair that is most susceptible to the effects of environmental conditions and cosmetic preparations and procedures. From the external surface inwards, the hair shaft comprises the cuticle, cortex, and medulla (Fig. 1.1b).

The Cuticle

The cuticle is the outermost layer of the hair shaft and is composed of the protein keratin. It protects the underlying cortex by providing a barrier to chemicals and water [2]. It consists of flat overlapping cells in a scale-like formation, with the proximal insertion firmly attached to the cortex and the distal free edges pointing toward the tip of the hair fiber (Fig. 1.2) [2, 3]. A healthy, intact cuticle has a smooth surface and low friction in the root to tip direction and contributes to the sheen associated with healthy hair. A damaged cuticle results in hair that is frizzy, dull, and prone to breakage.

Although the chemical composition of the cuticle is similar in all hair types, there are decreasing numbers of cuticular cell layers in Asian, Caucasian, and African hair [2, 4]. This relatively thinner cuticle layer in African hair contributes to a higher prevalence of hair breakage compared to Asian and Caucasian hair [2, 4, 5]. Additionally, cuticular cells become increasingly worn or absent in the root to tip direction in all hair types [6].

The outer aspect of the cuticle contains lipids (fatty acids, ceramides, and cholesterol) that contribute to the barrier function of the cuticle and promote the hydrophobicity and low friction of healthy hair [2–4, 7]. African hair has been shown to contain more total hair fiber lipids compared to Caucasian and Asian hair [7]. However, the use of alkaline chemical cosmetics that remove this lipid layer, such as anionic shampoos, sodium and lithium hydroxide, guanidine, and ammonium thioglycolate may damage the hair by disrupting barrier function and increasing penetration of water and other external materials into the hair fiber [2, 4, 7] (see Chaps. 2 and 7).

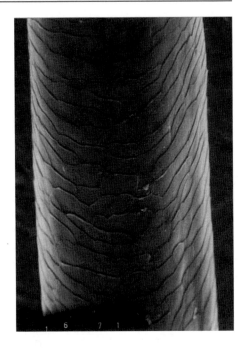

Fig. 1.2 Electron micrograph showing the overlapping, scale-like cells of the cuticle layer. (Reprinted from: Wolfram LJ. Human hair: a unique physicochemical composite. J Am Acad Dermatol. 2003;48(6 Suppl):S106-14, with permission from Elsevier)

The Cortex

The majority of the mass and the tensile strength of the hair shaft can be attributed to the cortex [8]. The cortex comprises keratin filaments and melanin granules, which determine hair color [2]. The keratin filaments are embedded in a cystine-rich matrix. Cystine is an amino acid that connects keratin proteins via many disulfide bonds [2, 9]. These disulfide bonds impart high mechanical strength to the hair and are altered during chemical treatments [8].

There is a strong adhesive layer between the cells of the cortex, known as the cell membrane complex (CMC). The CMC is vulnerable to cosmetic chemical hair treatments, such as bleaching, dyeing, straightening, and perming [4, 10, 11]. The CMC may even been disrupted during everyday grooming and shampooing, thus affecting the mechanical strength of the hair shaft [2, 4]. When the cuticle is damaged, the CMC can serve as a route of propagation of "split ends," which are longitudinal splits in the hair shaft [2, 4].

Cortical cells in human hair are divided into different regions termed orthocortex, paracortex, and mesocortex [8]. The distribution of these cell types is thought to be an important factor in determining curliness of the hair (see Curly Hair) [9, 12].

Cystine and Chemical Bonds in the Cortex

There is no difference in the cystine content of keratin proteins between African hair and that of other racial groups [13]. However, cosmetic chemical procedures, such as permanent hair straightening (relaxing), permanent waving, and bleaching of the hair, disrupt disulfide bonds in order to create these irreversible hairstyles. Cystine and the disulfide bonds it produces are also abundant in the cells of the cortex and [3, 9]. They are important to the tensile strength of the hair and are therefore important in the prevention of hair breakage. Cystine content is lower in damaged or weathered hair. African hair that has been permanently straightened (i.e., chemically relaxed) shows significantly lower cystine levels than untreated hair, suggesting an association between permanent straightening and hair damage [14].

In addition to disulfide bonds, keratin proteins are also linked by weaker bonds, such as hydrogen bonds, which can be easily disrupted by water to create temporary hair styles, e.g., using rollers on wet hair to create curls ("wet-setting") [2].

The Medulla

The medulla forms the porous, empty center of the hair fiber (Fig. 1.1b) [15]. It is not always present in human hairs, but is more likely to be found in coarser hair fibers with larger diameter, as is seen in gray hair and Asian hair [4, 16, 17]. The medulla contains structural proteins that are resistant to chemical treatment [16] but seems to contribute negligibly to the chemical and mechanical properties of the hair [2].

In summary, a healthy hair shaft has an intact, smooth cuticle with high lipid content from root to tip and a strong cortex with intact CMCs and many disulfide bonds. These basic building blocks of healthy hair are similar in all races/ethnicities, but are vulnerable to disruption by cosmetic products and styling practices. Significant changes in the disulfide and hydrogen bonds in keratin is crucial to nearly any modification to hair, including permanent curling/straightening procedures, bleaching, wet-setting, and even daily grooming procedures such as shampooing.

Anatomy of the Hair: Dermal Structures

The Inner and Outer Root Sheaths

In the dermis, the inner root sheath (IRS) surrounds the hair shaft cuticle layer (Fig. 1.1a). It is a rigid structure that is essential for proper hair shaft formation [18]. It serves as a guide to mold the hair shaft up to the level of the sebaceous gland, at which point the IRS disintegrates [19–21]. Early disintegration of the IRS has been associated with Central Centrifugal Cicatricial Alopecia (CCCA), a type of scarring hair loss seen almost exclusively in black women [22] (see Chap. 10). External to the IRS is the outer root sheath (ORS).

Sebaceous Glands

Conclusions from studies on racial differences in sebaceous gland size and activity are conflicting. Current opinion suggests that there are very few differences among different racial groups in this regard. However, in African hair and other curly hair types it is more difficult for sebum to make its way from the scalp down the hair shaft. Thus, curly hair types tend to be relatively dry and require regular application of cosmetic products to promote moisture retention.

Blood Supply
Studies on the racial differences of cutaneous blood supply have also shown conflicting results. However, it has been suggested that blood flow to the hair follicle in blacks is lower compared to whites, and this may contribute to the increased prevalence of scarring alopecia in black women [23].

Elastic Fibers
Differences in elastic fibers among racial groups have been reported. Black patients had fewer elastic fibers anchoring their hair follicles as compared to whites [24]. This observation may explain black patients' susceptibility to traction alopecia.

Physical Characteristics of the Hair

Growth Properties

The human hair follicle grows in a continuous cyclical pattern characterized by a period of growth (anagen) followed by involution (catagen) and resting (telogen) periods [19]. Each hair on the human scalp grows steadily at approximately 1 cm per month [3, 19]. Anagen is the growing phase that determines hair length and can last for 1–10 years (median of 3 years) [3, 19]. Catagen is much shorter than anagen and only lasts for approximately 3 weeks, during which metabolic activity slows as the hair bulb degenerates [2]. The telogen phase lasts approximately 3 months [19]. In this stage, growth has completely stopped and the base of the bulb atrophies [2]. As a new growth cycle begins, a new hair grows underneath the old hair in the same follicle and the old hair shaft is shed [3, 19] (Fig. 1.3). Approximately, 50–100 telogen hairs are shed daily [3].

At any given time, approximately 90 % of the hairs on the scalp are in anagen phase, and approximately 10–15 % of hairs are in telogen phase [3]. However in telogen effluvium, a common cause of non-scarring alopecia, there is an increase in the number of hairs in telogen phase which results in shedding of a larger than normal number of hairs. This is often a temporary condition that resolves over time without treatment.

No racial difference in the hair growth cycle or in the number of hairs in anagen and telogen phase has been found [23]. However, the average duration of the anagen phase decreases during the course of natural aging. Additionally, there are more hairs in the telogen phase (and therefore an increase in the subsequent hair shedding) in late summer and early autumn months [19]. These normal variations are important to consider when evaluating patients with alopecia.

Although there are no racial differences in the hair growth cycle, differences in the hair growth rate have been reported [23]. Studies have shown that African hair grows slower on average than Caucasian and Asian hair, with the latter ethnic group having the fastest growth rate of the three [23]. However, recent studies in individuals with straight hair have demonstrated that, regardless of race, individuals with larger diameter hair fibers have a faster growth rate. It is unclear if these results are generalizable to curly hair [23, 25].

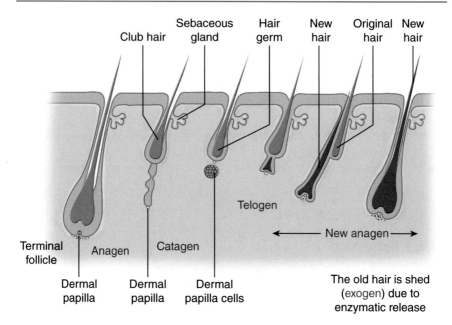

Fig. 1.3 The hair growth cycle

Porosity and Water Content

Hair is porous, meaning that it can absorb water from its environment. Humidity affects hair form and structure at the level of the hydrogen bonds [8]. Increase in ambient humidity significantly increases the water content of hair, causing swelling of the hair fibers and increased volume and frizz [8, 26] (see Chap. 8). This effect is accentuated in damaged hair [2, 4]. The water content of hair fibers has been shown to vary by race, with Caucasian hair having a higher water content than African and Asian hair [7, 27]. However, the water content of the hair is not synonymous with moisturization. The consumer perception of moisturization is related to subjective smoothness and softness and has not been shown to correlate with the water content of the hair.

Hair Shaft

Hair shape varies dramatically across African, Asian, and Caucasian hair types. Asian hair tends to be straight, and the cross-sectional area of the hair shaft is rounder and has the greatest diameter when compared to other races. The Caucasian hair shaft tends to have a diameter and cross-sectional shape that is intermediate between Asian and African hair, and Caucasian hair shows a wide range of curliness (Fig. 1.4) [28–30]. The cross-section of the African hair shaft has the most elliptical shape and its diameter varies throughout the hair shaft. It also shows the greatest

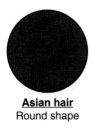

| **Asian hair** | **Caucasian hair** | **African hair** |
| Round shape | Slightly less round than asian hair | Oval or elliptical shape |

Fig. 1.4 Differences in the diameter and cross-sectional shape of Asian, Caucasian, and African hair

amount of hair shape variability, including differences in degree of ellipticity among people, among hairs from the same scalp, and even within the same hair shaft [28–30]. The African hair shaft is characterized by frequent twists along its longitudinal axis. The diameter of the hair shaft is smaller, and the hair may even appear flattened at the twisting points [4].

The African hair shaft is characterized by a very tightly coiled spring-like appearance. The narrow angles of the twists in curly African hair make it more susceptible to breakage [2]. During combing and grooming, African hair has been noted to have a significantly higher incidence of knotting and hair shaft breakage when compared to Caucasian and Asian hair. A higher incidence of structural damage, including full breaks, partial breaks, complex knots, and longitudinal splits, is also observed in African hair compared to Caucasians [5] (Fig. 1.5). This makes combing through the hair more traumatic to the hair fibers, especially when the hair is dry [27, 30]. Thus, frequent combing of very curly African hair is associated with increased frequency of hair breakage, and combing through wet hair is preferable to combing through dry hair [23, 27, 28, 30].

Hair Fragility

Hair strength depends on cuticle and cortex integrity and the amount of water in the hair fibers [2, 4]. Hair strength and integrity is significantly reduced by chemical procedures such as bleaching, dyeing, permanent straighteners, and permanent curls [2, 4, 31].

Since disulfide bonds have a major role in stabilizing the keratin structure, the inherent strength of hair shafts is related to both the quantity and distribution of cystine-rich proteins in the cortex and cuticle [3, 11]. Studies have proven that the quantity and distribution of cystine-rich proteins in African hair are similar to that of other races [3, 11]. Thus, there is no chemical evidence from this perspective that African hair is inherently weaker. Nonetheless, African hair has been shown to have a lower tensile strength and is less resistant to damage than Asian and Caucasian hair [29]. However, studies have shown that this apparent fragility of African hair is more attributable to physical damage rather than an inherent weakness in the structure of the African hair shaft [5, 11]. Additionally, African hair is generally tightly curled with twists and complex knots along the hair shaft, which makes it more susceptible to damage with daily grooming.

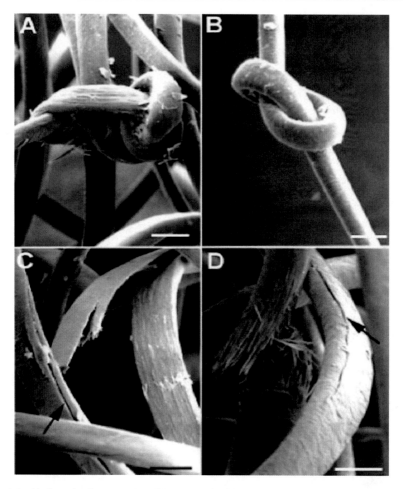

Fig. 1.5 (**a**) Complex knot seen in African hair. (**b**) Simple knot characteristic of knots seen in Caucasian hair. (**c, d**) Complex knots lead to longitudinal splits along the hair shaft. (Reprinted from: Khumalo NP, Doe PT, Dawber RP, Ferguson DJ. What is normal black African hair? A light and scanning electron-microscopic study. J Am Acad Dermatol. 2000;43(5 Pt 1):814-20, with permission from Elsevier)

The Science of Curly Hair

The mechanism of how natural curl develops is still unclear, but there are several theories regarding this phenomenon. Previously, the curliness of the hair shaft was believed to be determined by the shape of the hair follicle [19]. This theory has been disproven, and the current prevailing dogma suggests that hair curliness results from variations in the content and distribution of cortical cells [9, 14].

Curl Patterns

There is tremendous variability in hair curl patterns seen around the world, with significant overlap among people of different races. This variability and overlap renders describing curl patterns by race inaccurate. Hair curl types range from very straight to wavy to tightly curled (also called "kinky" or "coily") hair. Curls are often described subjectively but a few attempts have been made to create well-defined objective measurements of hair curliness.

In popular culture, curl patterns are classified according to a subjective classification system set forth by hairstylist Andre Walker in 1997. Hair is divided into the following categories: "Straight" (Type 1A–1C), "Wavy" (Type 2A–2C), "Curly" (Type 3A–3B), and "Kinky" (Type 4A–4B) [32] (Fig. 1.6a–d). This classification is

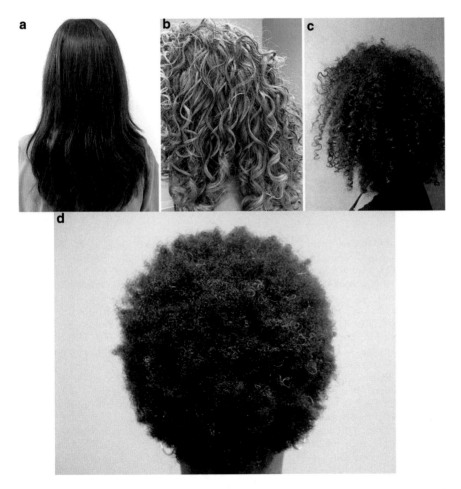

Fig. 1.6 Examples of hair curl types based on the Andre Walker classification system (**a**) Type 1 (straight) (**b**) Type 2 (wavy/curly hair) (**c**) Type 3 (curly) (**d**) Type 4 (kinky)

Table 1.1 Comparison of hair characteristics and curl types among different ethnic groups

Race	Appearance on cross section	Walker classification	Loussouarn classification	Growth rate (μm/day) [35]	Hair density (hairs/cm^2) [35]
African	Oval/elliptical	3A–4B	Type IV–VIII	280	161
Asian	Round	1A–2A	Type I–III	411	175
Caucasian	Intermediate between round and elliptical	1A–3A	Type I–IV	367	226

easy to use and widely accepted and has been adapted by consumers and the cosmetic industry (Table 1.1).

There have been several studies that sought to characterize hair curliness using objective measurements such as curve diameter and the number of waves and twists in the hair shaft [1, 33, 34] The most recent studies validated a classification system in which curl types are divided into eight patterns (Types I–VIII) [1, 33]. This system attempts to provide a way to more accurately describe curly hair without necessarily referring to ethnic origin. From Type I to Type VIII, the number of waves and twists increases, and the diameter of hair curls decreases. Based on this classification scheme, Asian hair is most often type II, Caucasian hair is most often types II and III, and African hair is most often types V to VII.

Including curl typing in the evaluation of patients' hair will facilitate better understanding of the properties of that individual's hair which can then inform hair management and cosmetic product recommendations (Table 1.1).

References

1. De la Mettrie R, Saint-Leger D, Loussouarn G, Garcel A, Porter C, Langaney A. Shape variability and classification of human hair: a worldwide approach. Hum Biol. 2007;79(3):265–81.
2. Robbins C. Chemical and physical behavior of human hair. 4th ed. New York: Springer; 2013.
3. Wolfram LJ. Human hair: a unique physicochemical composite. J Am Acad Dermatol. 2003;48(6 Suppl):S106–14.
4. Gavazzoni Dias MF. Hair cosmetics: an overview. Int J Trichol. 2015;7(1):2–15.
5. Khumalo NP, Doe PT, Dawber RP, Ferguson DJ. What is normal black African hair? A light and scanning electron-microscopic study. J Am Acad Dermatol. 2000;43(5 Pt 1):814–20.
6. Wei G, Bhushan B, Torgerson PM. Nanomechanical characterization of human hair using nanoindentation and SEM. Ultramicroscopy. 2005;105(1–4):248–66.
7. Marti M, Barba C, Manich AM, Rubio L, Alonso C, Coderch L. The influence of hair lipids in ethnic hair properties. Int J Cosmet Sci. 2016;38(1):77–84.
8. Araujo R, Fernandes M, Cavaco-Paulo A, Gomes A. Biology of human hair: know your hair to control it. Adv Biochem Eng Biotechnol. 2011;125:121–43.
9. Yang FC, Zhang Y, Rheinstadter MC. The structure of people's hair. Peer J. 2014;2, e619.
10. Robbins C, Scott C, Burnhurst J. A study of the causes of variation in the acid dye combining capacity of human hair. Text Res J. 1968;38:1130.
11. Dawber R. Hair: its structure and response to cosmetic preparations. Clin Dermatol. 1996;14(1):105–12.
12. Kajiura Y, Watanabe S, Itou T, Nakamura K, Iida A, Inoue K, et al. Structural analysis of human hair single fibres by scanning microbeam SAXS. J Struct Biol. 2006;155(3):438–44.

13. Khumalo NP, Dawber RP, Ferguson DJ. Apparent fragility of African hair is unrelated to the cystine-rich protein distribution: a cytochemical electron microscopic study. Exp Dermatol. 2005;14(4):311–4.
14. Khumalo NP, Stone J, Gumedze F, McGrath E, Ngwanya MR, de Berker D. 'Relaxers' damage hair: evidence from amino acid analysis. J Am Acad Dermatol. 2010;62(3):402–8.
15. Feughelman M. Mechanical properties and structure of alpha-keratin fibres: wool, human hair and related fibres. Sydney: UNSW Press; 1997.
16. Pierard-Franchimont C, Paquet P, Quatresooz P, Pierard GE. Mechanobiology and cell tensegrity: the root of ethnic hair curling? J Cosmet Dermatol. 2011;10(2):163–7.
17. Kamath Y, Weigmann H. Fractography of human hair. J Appl Polym Sci. 1982;27(10):3809–33.
18. Schlake T. Determination of hair structure and shape. Semin Cell Dev Biol. 2007;18(2):267–73.
19. Bernard BA. Hair shape of curly hair. J Am Acad Dermatol. 2003;48(6 Suppl):S120–6.
20. Sperling LC. Hair anatomy for the clinician. J Am Acad Dermatol. 1991;25(1 Pt 1):1–17.
21. Commo S, Bernard BA. Immunohistochemical analysis of tissue remodelling during the anagen-catagen transition of the human hair follicle. Br J Dermatol. 1997;137(1):31–8.
22. Sperling LC, Sau P. The follicular degeneration syndrome in black patients. 'Hot comb alopecia' revisited and revised. Arch Dermatol. 1992;128(1):68–74.
23. Lewallen R, Francis S, Fisher B, Richards J, Li J, Dawson T, et al. Hair care practices and structural evaluation of scalp and hair shaft parameters in African American and Caucasian women. J Cosmet Dermatol. 2015;14(3):216–23.
24. Montagna W, Carlisle K. The architecture of black and white facial skin. J Am Acad Dermatol. 1991;24(6):929–37.
25. Baque CS, Zhou J, Gu W, Collaudin C, Kravtchenko S, Kempf JY, et al. Relationships between hair growth rate and morphological parameters of human straight hair: a same law above ethnical origins? Int J Cosmet Sci. 2012;34(2):111–6.
26. Schueller R, Romanowski P. The science of reactive hair-care products. Cosmet Toilet. 1998;113:39–44.
27. Syed A, Kuhajda A, Ayoub H, Ahmad K, Frank E. African-American hair: its physical properties and differences relative to Caucasian hair. Cosmet Toilet. 1995;110:39–48.
28. Kamath Y, Hornby S, Weigmann H. Mechanical and fractographic behavior of negroid hair. J Soc Cosmet Chem. 1984;35:21–43.
29. Robbins C. The physical properties and cosmetic behavior of hair. New York: Springer; 1988.
30. Franbourg A, Hallegot P, Baltenneck F, Toutain C, Leroy F. Current research on ethnic hair. J Am Acad Dermatol. 2003;48(6 Suppl):S115–9.
31. Swift JA. The mechanics of fracture of human hair. Int J Cosmet Sci. 1999;21(4):227–39.
32. Robbins C, Reich C. Prediction of hair assembly characteristics from single-fiber properties. Part II. The relationship of fiber curvature, friction, stiffness, and diameter to combing behavior. J Soc Cosmet Chem. 1986;37:141–58.
33. A W. Andre talks hair! New York: Simon & Schuster; 1997.
34. Loussouarn G, Garcel AL, Lozano I, Collaudin C, Porter C, Panhard S, et al. Worldwide diversity of hair curliness: a new method of assessment. Int J Dermatol. 2007;46 Suppl 1:2–6.
35. Loussouarn G, El Rawadi C, Genain G. Diversity of hair growth profiles. Int J Dermatol. 2005;44(s1):6–9.

Part II

Aesthetic Modifications of Ethnic Hair

Chemical Modifications of Ethnic Hair

2

Alessandra Haskin, Ginette A. Okoye, and Crystal Aguh

Introduction

Hair is one of the few physical features that can be easily altered in its shape, color, and length. This chapter will discuss some of the methods used to esthetically modify the appearance of hair, with an emphasis on chemical processes commonly used in ethnic communities. This includes detailed descriptions of the processes involved in chemical relaxation, texturizing, and hair coloring, in addition to the potential deleterious effects of these chemical modifications.

Chemical Straightening

Chemical Relaxing

The use of chemical relaxers, also known as "perms," is arguably one of the most popular black hair care practices. Historically, black hair in its natural state was considered by many to be "unkempt" and socially unacceptable due to the societal norms and values of the time. In the early 1900s, Madame C.J. Walker introduced a method of hair straightening referred to as "hot combing," which

A. Haskin, B.A.
Howard University College of Medicine, 520 W St. NW, Washington, DC 20059, USA

G.A. Okoye, M.D. • C. Aguh, M.D. (✉)
Department of Dermatology, Johns Hopkins University School of Medicine,
5200 Eastern Avenue, Suite 2500, Baltimore, MD 21224, USA

© Springer International Publishing Switzerland 2017
C. Aguh, G.A. Okoye (eds.), *Fundamentals of Ethnic Hair*,
DOI 10.1007/978-3-319-45695-9_2

involved the use of oil-based pomades and heated metal combs to temporarily straighten the hair and increase the ease of combing and styling [1–3]. This technique quickly changed the practice of black hairstyling until a chance discovery by Garrett Augusta Morgan, a black tailor, led to the development of the first chemical relaxer [4]. While attempting to create a sewing machine lubricant, Morgan found that the liquid also straightened the fibers of wool cloth, and this effect was duplicated on the hair of a dog and Morgan's own curly hair [5]. In 1913, the first chemical relaxer was patented and sold as *G.A Morgan's hair refiner* [5]. The original formula, which consisted of rudimentary preparations of sodium hydroxide and starch, subsequently underwent numerous modifications and was officially introduced into the commercial market in the 1950s [6]. These alkaline-based chemical hair straighteners quickly revolutionized black hairstyling by providing a permanent method of straightening black hair. Continued advancements in product formulas led to the production of chemical relaxers marketed for at-home use, thereby increasing the accessibility of these products to more consumers.

It has been reported that at least 70 % of black women in the US have used chemical relaxers at least once in their lifetime [7, 8]. Although these products have traditionally been very popular in the black community, more women are now opting for natural, "chemical-free" hairstyling practices (see Chap. 8). This has led to a recent decline in the use of chemical relaxers. Reports suggest that chemical relaxer sales have declined by 26 % since 2008 [9]. Despite these statistics, a significant number of individuals from various ethnic backgrounds continue to use chemical relaxers, with many viewing this practice as a lifestyle preference that increases the versatility of hairstyling and improves manageability.

The process of chemical relaxation or lanthionization involves the permanent alteration of the hair's keratin molecules, which are composed of strong bonds (disulfide bonds) and weak bonds (hydrogen bonds, van der Waals forces, and ionic bonds) (see Chap. 1) [1]. Disruption of disulfide bonds, which maintain the coiled shape of ethnic hair, results in permanent alteration of the hair's texture. Chemical relaxers function by altering the amino acid compositions of keratin by replacing cysteine with lanthionine and irreversibly cleaving disulfide bonds, which resets the hair shaft into a straighter from [10–12].

There are many different chemical relaxers on the market including emulsions of sodium, potassium, lithium, or guanidine hydroxide [1, 10]. These highly alkaline chemicals facilitate opening of the hair cuticle scales by swelling the hair shaft, which allows for penetration of the straightening agents into the cortex [1, 13]. Based on the active ingredient, chemical relaxers can be separated into two categories: lye and no-lye relaxers.

The active ingredient in lye relaxers is sodium hydroxide, which results in a very alkaline pH of 13–14 [14]. Lye relaxers have been purported to be less drying and damaging to the hair because they do not leave mineral deposits, which impede moisture absorption, on the hair shaft [15]. However, they are more irritating to the scalp and can quickly cause chemical burns. Therefore, they have been traditionally recommended for salon use only [15].

No-lye relaxers typically contain guanidine or lithium hydroxide and are available in mix or no-mix formulations [14, 15]. Mix formulations require the mixture of calcium hydroxide (relaxer base) and guanidine carbonate (activator) to create the active ingredient, guanidine hydroxide (Table 2.1) (Fig. 2.1) [2, 6, 14]. This formulation typically has a pH of 11–13. This mixture must be used on the same day to avoid chemical alteration, as guanidine hydroxide does not remain stable for an extended period of time [2, 15]. No-mix formulations contain lithium hydroxide and do not require mixing of relaxer components before use [15]. No-lye relaxers are less irritating to the scalp; however, they leave behind dulling calcium deposits that increase the brittleness of the hair [14, 15]. Chelating shampoos are often required for effective removal of these deposits [14, 15]. It is important to note that because no-lye relaxers are associated with

Table 2.1 Lye vs. no-lye chemical relaxers

Lye chemical relaxers	No-lye chemical relaxers
• Sodium hydroxide	• Guanidine, lithium, or potassium hydroxide
• Professional application recommended	• Generally considered safe for at-home use
• More likely to irritate the scalp	• Less likely to irritate the scalp
• Less likely to leave behind mineral deposits that can leave hair dry and brittle	• More likely to leave behind mineral deposits

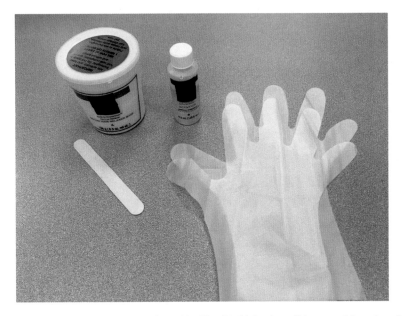

Fig. 2.1 Components of a no-lye relaxer kit. The liquid "activator" is poured into the tub of "relaxer base" and mixed with the spatula immediately before application

less burning or stinging, patients may be tempted to leave these relaxers in the hair for longer periods of time, allowing for increased disulfide bond breakage and straighter hair [15]. However, this may result in dry, overprocessed hair that is prone to breakage [15]. No-lye relaxers are more accessible for general consumer use and can be found in most retail stores.

The process of chemical relaxing involves four steps:

1. *Processing*: The processing phase begins with the application of a protective "base coat" of petroleum jelly to the scalp, hairline, and ears. The hair is then parted into sections and the chemical relaxer is applied using a small brush or comb [2] (Fig. 2.2). *After the relaxer has been applied to the hair shaft, a comb is used to manually straighten the hair into its anticipated final orientation.* The relaxer is typically left in the hair for 10–20 min. However, the exact length of time depends on the manufacturer's instructions [11]. It should be noted that these highly alkaline agents will digest the hair if left on for too long; therefore, this aspect of the process has to be carefully timed and monitored [11].

2. *Neutralizing*: Once the hair has been sufficiently processed, the relaxer is thoroughly rinsed out with warm water followed by a neutralizing shampoo, which stops the chemical reaction of the relaxer [2]. Neutralizing shampoos (pH 4.5–6) restore the normal pH of the hair and facilitate the reformation of disulfide bonds in their new *straightened* position [11].

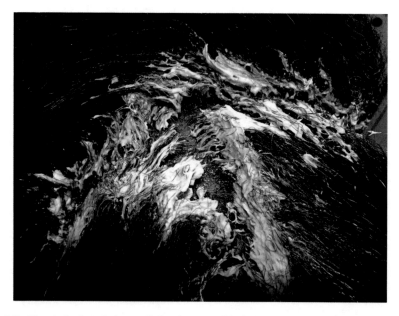

Fig. 2.2 Chemical relaxer being applied to the roots of the hair to permanently straighten the curly "new growth"

3. *Conditioning*: The chemical relaxing process opens the hair cuticle leaving it unable to retain moisture and increasing its susceptibility to breakage; therefore, a conditioner is typically applied to the hair after the relaxing treatment [11].
4. *Retouching*: Patients should have at least 6 weeks of hair growth to minimize likelihood of applying relaxer to previously treated hair [10]. Since chemical relaxers lead to permanent straightening, reapplication should only be performed on the unrelaxed roots to avoid over-processing and breakage of previously treated hair.

Texturizing

Texturizing is a permanent chemical straightening process very similar to chemical relaxing; however, it is formulated to "loosen" the natural curl pattern of the hair instead of completely straightening it. Initially marketed towards men to create sleek, "wavy" hairstyles, these products have recently gained popularity among women as well.

Texturizers and relaxers are often marketed as completely different hair care products, with texturizers sometimes advertised as "natural" or "safer" alternatives to chemical relaxers. However, it should be emphasized that most texturizers contain active ingredients identical to those found in chemical relaxers, specifically sodium or guanidine hydroxide. Both products permanently straighten the hair via irreversible cleavage of disulfide bonds within the hair's keratin molecules. The primary difference between these processes is that texturizers are left on the hair for shorter periods of time, which results in less disulfide bond breakage and more retention of the hair's natural curl pattern. Some texturizers contain ammonium thioglycolate as the active agent, which is a less alkaline chemical straightener that selectively weakens the hair's disulfide bonds instead of breaking them, resulting in more loosely coiled strands [13].

Texturizers are applied to the hair using the same techniques as chemical relaxers; however, they are typically left on the hair for no more than 5–10 min. The product is then rinsed out and the hair is washed with a neutralizing shampoo. Similar to chemical relaxers, this process must be repeated but should only be applied to new growth. The timing of reapplication varies depending on hair growth and texture; however, many individuals repeat this process every 3–5 months. One of the main disadvantages of texturizers is the difficulty in maintaining a uniform texture with each reapplication. If the product is applied to previously processed hair, those strands will be completely straightened, resulting in an uneven mix of coiled and straightened hair. As a result, texturizers produce more favorable results when applied to shorter hair, in which it is easier to maintain a uniform curl pattern.

"Texlaxing" is a technique used to achieve texturized hair but involves the use of traditional chemical relaxers (instead of products labeled as texturizers). The product is left in the hair for a shorter length of time, thus deliberately "under processing" the hair [15]. This can also be accomplished by diluting the consistency of chemical relaxers by adding oils or conditioners, which prolong the processing time for disulfide bond breakage [15].

Texturizers are considered by some to be relatively safer than chemical relaxers because their active ingredients are in contact with the hair for shorter periods of time, enabling the hair to retain much of its natural, unprocessed strength [15]. However, it should be noted that the hair damage associated with chemical relaxers can also be caused by texturizers.

Hair Damage Associated with Chemical Straightening

During the process of chemical straightening, the rearrangement of hydrogen and disulfide bonds results in the formation of new bonds that are weaker due to the overall loss of sulfur, which increases the fragility of the hair shaft [14]. The foul smell described by many patients during the relaxing process is due to disulfide bond breakage of sulfur-containing amino acids, resulting in the loss of free sulfur from the hair shaft and weakening of the protein structure [12]. The link between hair fragility and chemical relaxing was demonstrated by Khumalo et al., who performed biochemical analysis of natural hair, symptomatic (brittle) relaxed hair, and asymptomatic relaxed hair in African women [16]. Their findings indicated that the content of cystine, a sulfur-containing amino acid, was decreased in chemically relaxed hair (both symptomatic and asymptomatic) compared to natural hair and that these reduced levels were similar to those observed in the genetic hair fragility disorder, trichothiodystrophy [16]. The results of this study also indicated that the cystine content was lower in distal hair compared to the proximal sections of the same hair shaft, suggesting that distal hair was more likely to have been repeatedly exposed to chemical relaxers [16]. This finding highlights the importance of only treating new growth when retouching chemically relaxed hair. Other side effects of chemical relaxers can include scalp irritation, chemical burns (Fig. 2.3), post-inflammatory hypopigmentation/hyperpigmentation, trichoptilosis (split ends), and tangling (distal acquired trichorrhexis nodosa) [11]. The association between the use of chemical relaxers and the development of scarring alopecia has long been hypothesized, but there are currently no studies definitively implicating this practice as a causative factor [17]. However, the misuse of chemical relaxers and subsequent scalp inflammation is considered to be at least an exacerbating risk factor for scarring alopecia [17].

Hair Coloring Techniques

Hair coloring is a practice used by both men and women and involves many different techniques and coloring agents [2]. Hair dyes are classified according to the depth of penetration into the hair shaft, which determines how long the color will remain on the hair [13].

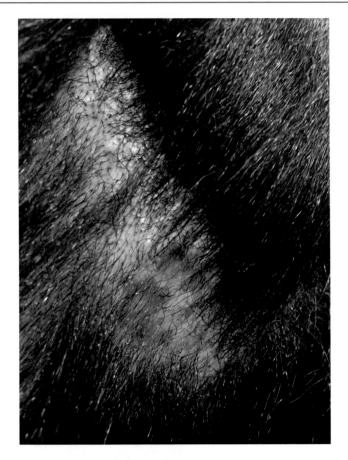

Fig. 2.3 Chemical burn on the scalp from a relaxer

Temporary Hair Dyes

Temporary hair dyes consist of acidic textile dyes that are water soluble and possess a high molecular weight [18, 19]. They are named for their ability to be removed after a single shampooing [2]. These large molecules are unable to penetrate the cuticle and are instead temporarily deposited on the surface layers until they are washed off [2, 19]. Temporary dyes are formulated as rinses, gels, mousses, and sprays and are primarily used to remove unwanted tones, add highlights, or subtly color the hair [20]. Rinses are applied after shampooing and immediately rinsed, while gels, mousses, and sprays are applied to towel-dried hair and left in for a specified amount of time [2]. When applied to chemically treated hair, the effects of temporary dyes are longer lasting because chemically treated hair is more porous, allowing for deeper penetration of the dye [2]. These products are generally considered safe as most are hypoallergenic and do not induce damage to the hair shaft [20]. Temporary dyes have the potential to rub off the hair shaft and on to clothing, especially when the hair becomes wet due to rain or perspiration [18].

Semipermanent Hair Dyes

Semipermanent dyes are composed of low molecular weight coal tar dyes and may contain hydrogen peroxide, resorcinol, and para-dyes such as diamines, aminophenols, and phenols [2, 13]. Their smaller molecular weight allows for shallow penetration into the cortex, resulting in color that typically lasts through 6–8 shampoos [2]. Semipermanent dyes are formulated as lotions and mousses and are applied to wet, shampooed hair for 10–40 min before being rinsed out [2]. These products cannot lighten the hair color, but can usually darken the hair by up to three tones [2]. Semipermanent dyes can cover up to 30 % of gray hair and are sometimes used to add shine and increase the vibrancy of the natural hair color [13, 20].

Demi-Permanent Hair Dyes

Demi-permanent dyes are replacing semipermanent dyes on the market because they are longer lasting, usually remaining through 10–12 shampoos [18]. Similar to semipermanent dyes, they also contain hydrogen peroxide, resorcinol, and para-dyes [13]. Demi-permanent dyes are considered to be gentler on the hair compared to permanent dyes since they do not contain ammonia or ethanolamine. Instead, they contain monoethanolamine to facilitate penetration of the coloring agents into the hair shaft [13, 21]. They also contain a lower concentration of hydrogen peroxide (2 %) compared to that of permanent dyes (6 %) [13]. These dyes are typically used to add red highlights to brown hair and can also be used to give the hair a burgundy hue [18]. They can cover up to 40–50 % of gray hair and do not lighten the hair color [13, 20]. These dyes also minimize the color difference between dyed hair and new hair growth, which can be drastic in permanently dyed hair [20].

Permanent Hair Dyes

Permanent hair dyes are the most prominent hair dyes on the market due to their ability to lighten darker hair and to cover any amount of gray hair [13]. Permanent hair dyes can include natural vegetable dyes and synthetic dyes [22]. The most commonly used natural dye is henna, also known as Lawsone, which is produced from the dried leaves of the Egyptian privet plant and colors the hair with an orange-red pigment (see Chap. 12) [22]. More recently, "compound henna" has become available, in which henna is combined with metallic salts to provide a wider range of colors [18]. Henna has also been combined with paraphenylenediamines (PPDs) to create a darker color. Other natural dyes can be extracted from nutgall, brazilwood, or logwood and are often used in Asian countries to blacken graying hair [2, 23]. One of the major disadvantages of using natural hair dyes is the limited color range and difficulty in predicting the intensity of color. Therefore, most consumers prefer the use of synthetic dyes [2].

Synthetic dyes contain paraphenylenediamines (PPDs) which are derivatives of coal tar and synthetic aniline dyes [22]. These hair dyes are water soluble and have a small molecular weight, which allows for deeper penetration into the hair shaft [22]. Similar to chemical relaxers, permanent dyes require an alkaline pH to open the cuticle scales and allow pigment to reach the cortex [13]. Most permanent dye preparations contain ammonia to increase the pH; however, some products are marketed as "ammonia free" and instead contain ethanolamine to achieve the same effect [13]. These solutions also contain surfactants, solvents, thickeners, antioxidants, and metal chelating agents which prolong their shelf life [2]. Conditioners are also sometimes added to reduce resultant hair damage [2]. Permanent dyes are available as liquids, creams, or gels and all forms must be mixed with hydrogen peroxide (packaged separately) prior to application [22]. The dye mixture is applied to dry, unwashed hair and left in for 20–40 min and then rinsed off with water [2].

The process of permanent hair coloring involves an oxidation reaction, which relies on three major components: primary intermediates, couplers, and oxidants [2]. Primary intermediates are para-dyes such as PPD, *para*-toluenediamine, and *para*-aminophenol, which undergo oxidation to produce color [2, 13]. Hydrogen peroxide, the oxidant in this reaction, oxidizes the primary intermediates [2, 22]. Couplers (phenols, *meta*-aminophenols, and *meta*-diaminobenzenes) react with the products of oxidation to produce indo dyes, which are larger, insoluble molecules that become trapped within the cortex [2, 22]. These newly formed molecules are too large to pass through the cuticle, which is why they cannot be washed out [22]. Variation in color selection is determined by the concentrations of hydrogen peroxide, primary intermediates, and couplers in the dye preparation [20]. The desired color determines the strength of hydrogen peroxide required [22]. Covering dyes tint the hair to a shade darker than the original color and tend to contain 20 vol. (6 %) hydrogen peroxide, while lightening dyes tint the hair to a shade lighter than the original color and require 30 vol. (9 %) hydrogen peroxide to be effective [22]. The hair should always be conditioned after this process, as the alkaline dye induces cuticular swelling that must be reversed to prevent excessive damage to the hair [18]. Although these dying products are labeled as "permanent," the color molecules can be extracted from the hair shaft with frequent washing and the use of harsh, sulfate-based shampoos [18]. Therefore, sulfate-free shampoos or mild surfactant shampoos formulated specifically for color-treated hair should be used to minimize color loss (see Chap. 7) [15, 18]. Re-dying is necessary every 2–3 months depending on the speed of new hair growth [20].

An additional step in this process is required for those who wish to achieve a hair color significantly lighter than their natural or baseline color [2, 23]. The hair must first be bleached using a solution containing hydrogen peroxide and boosters such as ammonium or potassium persulfate [23]. Once the hair is bleached to the desired shade, a dye can be applied to achieve the final color [2].

Hair Bleaching

Bleaching is a process that permanently lightens the shade of the hair via oxidation of melanin in the cortex, specifically eumelanin and pheomelanin [22]. The primary method of hair bleaching involves the use of alkaline solutions of up to 12 % hydrogen peroxide, which is the highest strength that can be safely used on the hair [2, 22]. Hair bleaching products are typically applied to dry unwashed hair, as sebum minimizes scalp irritation [18]. Proper technique requires that the solution be applied to the hair ends first to facilitate even coloring as the bleaching reaction occurs most rapidly near the scalp due to the presence of body heat [18]. Darker hair requires longer bleaching times, and red hair is more difficult to bleach than brown hair [2]. Serial bleaching of black hair goes through a series of color stages: black to brown to red to orange to yellow to pale yellow to white [22]. After the bleaching solution is left on the hair for the appropriate duration of time, it is removed by washing the hair with a low surfactant acidic pH shampoo, which minimizes damage by reversing the hair shaft swelling induced by the alkaline bleaching solutions [18]. These products are frequently used in combination with permanent dyes and toners to enhance the final color [23].

Unexpected results such as reddish or "brassy overtones" occur in brown hair that contains red undertones [20]. This phenomenon occurs because the pheomelanin responsible for reddish pigments is more resistant to removal by peroxide bleaching agents compared to eumelanin [20]. This "brassy" color typically appears 1–2 weeks after the bleaching procedure, as permanent dye molecules are removed from the hair shaft with shampooing [20]. This can be corrected by using a higher volume of hydrogen peroxide solution to completely remove the pheomelanin [20]. However, this will exacerbate the weakening of the hair by stripping additional protein [20]. Patients should select a darker shade closer to their natural hair color to avoid this problem [20].

Hair Dyes and Allergic Reactions

The primary agent in hair dyes responsible for allergic and irritant contact dermatitis is PPD [21]. This reaction is often characterized by pruritus and scalp erythema, with associated facial edema and eye swelling in severe cases [18]. All hair dye manufacturers recommend testing for the possibility of an allergic reaction by applying a small amount of the dye to a localized area of the scalp prior to use on the entire scalp [18]. Permanent and semipermanent dyes pose the highest risk of contact dermatitis, while temporary dyes pose the lowest risk [18]. Interestingly, African American patients have been shown to exhibit higher rates of sensitization to PPDs compared to Caucasian patients [24]. Boosters such as ammonium persulfate or potassium sulfate are frequently added to hair bleaching solutions and are also potential sources of allergic contact dermatitis [20]. The persulfate salts may also trigger immediate reactions such as rhinitis, asthma, and contact urticaria [21].

Hair Damage Associated with Hair Coloring Techniques

Hair coloring, especially permanent and semipermanent processing can cause damage by disrupting the hair's cuticle integrity and protein structure [15]. These processes can lead to hair fiber swelling, cuticle detachment, and possible complete exposure of the cortex [15]. The alkaline ingredients in hair dye formulations cause cuticle damage by removing the natural cuticle lipid 18-methyl eicosanoic acid (18-MEA), which contributes to the hydrophobicity of hair fibers [13].

The process of bleaching is extremely damaging to the hair shaft as the involved oxidation reaction destroys some of the disulfide bonds within keratin molecules [2]. Specifically, bleaching causes degradation of the amino acids tyrosine, threonine, and methionine along with a loss of 15–25 % of disulfide bonds and 45 % of cystine bonds within the hair shaft [20]. This increases the porosity of the cuticle, resulting in increased fragility [21]. Bleached hair often has a different texture and is more susceptible to humidity [2]. This is because bleached hair is more porous due to loss of cuticular scale, resulting in increased water absorption, but poor moisture retention [18].

The previously described hair damage is often even more extreme in hair that has been both chemically straightened and permanently colored [15]. This is because both chemical processes work by breaching the cuticular layers and altering the hair's protein structure [15]. The combination of bleaching and chemical relaxing leaves the hair severely damaged and unable to withstand the trauma of routine grooming, resulting in hair that breaks at its exit point from the scalp [18].

If patients insist on permanently dyeing their chemically relaxed hair, it is very important that the dyeing procedure be performed at least 10–14 days after the straightening procedure to avoid an undesirable hair color and excessive damage to the hair shaft [15, 20]. Coloring chemically relaxed hair sooner than this recommended time frame can result in irreparable damage to the hair with a drastic increase in porosity and subsequent breakage [15]. It has been suggested that demipermanent dyes are safer than permanent dyes for use on chemically treated hair. Demi-permanent dyes do not contain ammonia or ethanolamine and are therefore less likely to induce the same amount of cuticular scale opening and hair breakage

Table 2.2 Key points to minimize damage from hair coloring techniques

- Hair should not be lightened or darkened by more than 3 shades from the natural/baseline color
- Hair lightening and bleaching should be discouraged as these techniques are more damaging, compared to hair darkening
- Application of temporary hair dyes is the safest technique of hair coloring
- If patients insist on coloring chemically straightened hair, the use of demi-permanent dye instead of permanent dye is recommended
- When coloring chemically straightened hair, the straightening procedure should be performed first, followed by the coloring procedure at least 14 days later
- Chemically processed hair should not be bleached
- Prolong the interval between hair dying sessions to minimize frequent exposure to dye preparations and subsequent hair damage
- Always condition the hair after and between coloring sessions
- Always test hair dyes before complete application to avoid allergic and irritant contact dermatitis
- Decrease the frequency of thermal straightening on color-treated hair as these practices degrade the hair cuticle causing the color to become dull over time

[13]. Table 2.2 summarizes important recommendations to minimize damage associated with hair coloring.

References

1. Tanus A, Oliveira CC, Villarreal DJ, Sanchez FA, Dias MF. Black women's hair: the main scalp dermatoses and aesthetic practices in women of African ethnicity. An Bras Dermatol. 2015;90(4):450–65.
2. Bolduc C, Shapiro J. Hair care products: waving, straightening, conditioning, and coloring. Clin Dermatol. 2001;19(4):431–6.
3. Callender VD, McMichael AJ, Cohen GF. Medical and surgical therapies for alopecias in black women. Dermatol Ther. 2004;17(2):164–76.
4. Aryiku SA, Salam A, Dadzie OE, Jablonski NG. Clinical and anthropological perspectives on chemical relaxing of afro-textured hair. J Eur Acad Dermatol Venereol. 2015;29(9):1689–95.
5. Obukowho P. History and evolution of hair relaxers. In: Hair relaxers science, design and application. Portland: Allured; 2012.
6. de Sa Dias TC, Baby AR, Kaneko TM, Robles Velasco MV. Relaxing/straightening of Afro-ethnic hair: historical overview. J Cosmet Dermatol. 2007;6(1):2–5.
7. Burrall BA. Ethnic skin: a spectrum of issues. 2006. Available from: http://www.medscape.org/viewarticle/529349.
8. Wise LA, Palmer JR, Reich D, Cozier YC, Rosenberg L. Hair relaxer use and risk of uterine leiomyomata in African-American women. Am J Epidemiol. 2012;175(5):432–40.
9. Hair relaxer sales decline 26% over the past five years. 2013. Available from: http://www.mintel.com/press-centre/beauty-and-personal-care/hairstyle-trends-hair-relaxer-sales-decline.
10. McMichael AJ. Ethnic hair update: past and present. J Am Acad Dermatol. 2003;48(6 Suppl):S127–33.
11. Quinn CR, Quinn TM, Kelly AP. Hair care practices in African American women. Cutis. 2003;72(4):280–2, 285–9.
12. Draelos ZD. Commentary: healthy hair and protein loss. J Am Acad Dermatol. 2010;62(3):409–10.
13. Gavazzoni Dias MF. Hair cosmetics: an overview. Int J Trichol. 2015;7(1):2–15.

14. Crawford K, Hernandez C. A review of hair care products for black individuals. Cutis. 2014;93(6):289–93.
15. Davis-Sivasothy A. The science of black hair: a comprehensive guide to textured hair care. Stafford: Saja Publishing; 2011.
16. Khumalo NP, Stone J, Gumedze F, McGrath E, Ngwanya MR, de Berker D. 'Relaxers' damage hair: evidence from amino acid analysis. J Am Acad Dermatol. 2010;62(3):402–8.
17. Gathers RC, Lim HW. Central centrifugal cicatricial alopecia: past, present, and future. J Am Acad Dermatol. 2009;60(4):660–8.
18. Draelos ZD. Hair care: an illustrated dermatologic handbook. London: Taylor & Francis; 2005.
19. Franca-Stefoni SA, Dario MF, Sa-Dias TC, Bedin V, de Almeida AJ, Baby AR, et al. Protein loss in human hair from combination straightening and coloring treatments. J Cosmet Dermatol. 2015;14(3):204–8.
20. Draelos ZD. Cosmetics: an overview. Curr Probl Dermatol. 1995;7(2):45–64.
21. Guerra-Tapia A, Gonzalez-Guerra E. Hair cosmetics: dyes. Actas Dermosifiliogr. 2014;105(9):833–9.
22. Gray J. Hair care and hair care products. Clin Dermatol. 2001;19(2):227–36.
23. Harrison S, Sinclair R. Hair colouring, permanent styling and hair structure. J Cosmet Dermatol. 2003;2(3–4):180–5.
24. Deleo VA, Taylor SC, Belsito DV, Fowler JF, Jr., Fransway AF, Maibach HI, et al. The effect of race and ethnicity on patch test results. J Am Acad Dermatol. 2002;46(2 Suppl Understanding):S107–12.

Thermal Modifications of Ethnic Hair

3

Alessandra Haskin, Crystal Aguh, and Ginette A. Okoye

Thermal Straightening

Since the era of the Ancient Egyptians, men and women have used thermal devices to manipulate and straighten the texture of curly hair [1]. Early hair straightening techniques involved the use of crude and dangerous materials until the 1900s when Madam C.J. Walker introduced and popularized a more advanced thermal straightening method into the commercial market [1–3]. This temporary hair straightening technique, typically referred to as "pressing" or "hot combing," involved the use of heated metal combs and oil-based pomades to straighten the texture of ethnic hair [2–4]. This process became widely popular among black women and rapidly changed the practice of black hairstyling due to its ability to increase the ease of everyday combing and promote versatility in hairstyling. Many patients begin thermal styling at a very young age, as some deem it to be safer than chemical styling for young children (Table 3.1). Despite the advent of "permanent" hair straightening techniques such as chemical relaxers, thermal hair straightening is still used today.

Thermal hair straightening involves the application of heat to temporarily straighten the hair. This is achieved by modifying hydrogen bonds in a process called keratin hydrolysis [3, 4]. This process is temporary; exposure to water or

A. Haskin, B.A.
Howard University College of Medicine, 520 W St. NW, Washington, DC 20059, USA

C. Aguh, M.D. • G.A. Okoye, M.D. (✉)
Department of Dermatology, Johns Hopkins University School of Medicine,
5200 Eastern Avenue, Suite 2500, Baltimore, MD 21224, USA

© Springer International Publishing Switzerland 2017
C. Aguh, G.A. Okoye (eds.), *Fundamentals of Ethnic Hair*,
DOI 10.1007/978-3-319-45695-9_3

Table 3.1 Patient Perspective

There are those "firsts" in life that you just don't forget—first kiss, first alcoholic drink, and first concert. Well, I also remember the first time I got my hair done at a salon. I was three. Now, before you scoff at the thought of a 3-year-old in a hair salon, let me assure you that I wasn't getting my hair done at a salon as a 3-year-old because I was spoiled or in any kind of beauty pageant; no, I was getting my hair done at a salon as a 3-year-old because my mother couldn't do it. No, my mom's not white, or Native American, or Latina, or Asian—she was just born with a very different grade of hair than I was blessed with. But this would confuse me as a very young child—if my mom looks like that, why do I look like this? Often, as a little girl, I would ask my mom if she were "Spanish" because her fair skin and straight, slightly curled hair looked more like that of a Latina than other black women I saw, or, even my own skin and hair. When I was three, I didn't yet understand the various shades, textures, and phenotypes that comprised blackness
At any rate, there I was, barely out of toddlerhood, at a salon getting my hair done. I remember watching my mother first getting her hair washed at the shampoo bowl. I didn't quite understand why she closed her eyes as the hairdresser massaged her scalp with shampoo and water, but I immediately knew that it would be proper to do the same thing. So as my stylist motioned me toward the bowl, I sat up as high as I could, leaned back, and closed my eyes as she, too, massaged my scalp with shampoo and water. Afterward, the stylist combed my hair out, taking my head with the comb as she pulled her arm out with the first full strokes. I quickly learned to keep my head upright and resist the urge to be pulled back with every stroke of the brush lest I look weak. "Good, you aren't tenderheaded," the stylist remarked more so as a threat than a compliment
As the stylist rolled my hair in tiny rollers, I fell deeper and deeper into boredom; I glanced at my mother who was also getting her hair rolled, and she gave me a reassuring nod. I was too young to fully comprehend that this would soon become a rite of passage, but somehow I understood that I needed to "act like a big girl." I joined my mother along the row of dryer stations, sitting under the heat blast for what seemed like an eternity. At this point, I just wanted to go home to watch my beloved Punky Brewster. But finally, finally, joy cometh after my stylist unfurled those several multicolored curlers, and I watched with childish astonishment as my locks—formerly a mere kinky mass of puffy—were now transformed into a cascade of silky ringlets
For the first time in my short life, my hair matched my mom's. My first experience had seemed an epic ordeal, but the end result was worth the process if it meant that I could feel like my mother's daughter

moisture will cause the hydrogen bonds to return to their original state, resulting in reversion of the hair to its natural curl pattern [5]. Currently, there are a variety of techniques used to thermally straighten hair.

Thermal Straightening and Styling Techniques

Hot Combing

Hot combing was the first thermal straightening method to become widely popular in the US. It involves the use of stainless steel or brass combs that are heated using household stoves or specially designed heating stoves that fit around the hot comb, called marcel stoves (Fig. 3.1) [5–7]. "Pressing" is a traditional thermal straightening practice in which the hair is

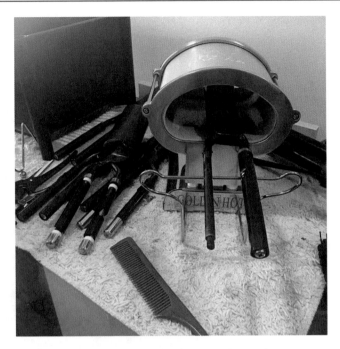

Fig. 3.1 Marcel stove, a specially designed stove for heating hot combs

washed and dried and an oil or petrolatum-based ointment is then applied to the hair, which softens and prepares the hair for straightening and helps protect the scalp from exposure to elevated temperatures [7]. The hot comb, typically heated to 300–500 °F, is then pulled through the hair from roots to ends resulting in significantly straighter hair. This process needs to be repeated every 1–2 weeks since normal perspiration and environmental humidity will cause reversion to the hair's natural curl pattern [5]. Although hot combs are still in use today, advancements in thermal straightening techniques have led to the development of more efficient thermal tools such as flat irons.

Flat Ironing

Flat irons, which consist of two electrically heated, smooth metal plates, have largely replaced hot combs in the practice of thermal hair straightening. They allow for better temperature control and are therefore easier and safer to use. Flat irons work best on hair that has been dried and partially straightened with a blow-dryer. The hair to be straightened is placed between the two metals plates which are then pressed together and moved downward along the hair shaft from root to tip (Fig. 3.2). An updated pressing technique called the "silk press" involves the use of flat irons and products containing silicones, such as dimethicone and cyclomethicone, which are applied prior to heat application to create a lighter, less weighed down, straightened look compared to the traditional press [8].

Fig. 3.2 Flat ironing for
thermal straightening. The
hair to be straightened is
placed between the two
metals plates which are
then pressed together and
moved downward along
the hair shaft from root to
tip

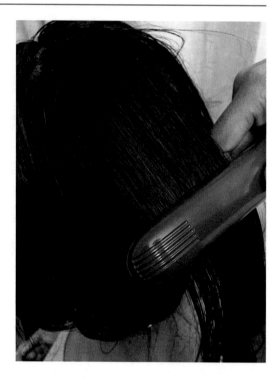

Most modern flat irons contain metal plates that are coated with thermal barrier materials such as ceramic or titanium, which promote thermal stability [6]. These materials also reduce friction during the thermal straightening process, which helps to maintain a smooth cuticular surface, thereby reducing hair damage and breakage [6]. Advances in the manufacturing of thermal styling tools have led to the development of pure ceramic flat irons and tourmaline (mineral) flat irons [6]. Manufacturers claim that these materials can have beneficial effects on the hair by emitting negative ions and infrared radiation, which are purported to help infuse moisture and increase the speed of styling [6, 8]. However, these claims have not yet been supported in the scientific literature.

Curling irons are similar hairstyling tools that are typically made of the same materials; however, they consist of round metal barrels of various sizes and are used to create the look of curled styles in straightened hair (Figs. 3.3 and 3.4).

Blow-Drying

Another frequently used tool for thermal straightening is the blow-dryer, which is a handheld tool that accelerates the process of drying wet hair and facilitates straightening by blowing high speed hot air over the hair shaft. Hooded dryers are another thermal styling tool that function similar to handheld blow-dryers. However, in hooded dryers, the hot air is emitted from a vented hard plastic

Fig. 3.3 "Barrel" type of curling iron

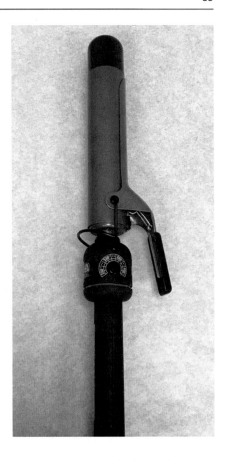

helmet that sits above the patient's head (Fig. 3.5). Patients typically apply rollers or wrap the hair in a circular motion around the head to effectively "set" the hair shafts in a straighter orientation, prior to drying the hair under a hooded dryer (Fig. 3.6). "Blowout" styles are achieved by using a large round brush while simultaneously blow-drying the hair. Using medium heat, the brush is run through the hair from root to tip to create a straightened look with loose curls at the end (Fig. 3.7a, b).

Hair Damage Associated with Thermal Straightening and Styling

The elevated temperatures of thermal styling tools can disrupt the protein linkages that maintain the strength of the hair shaft [8]. Healthy hair burns at 451.4 °F (233 °C), while previously damaged hair can burn at much lower temperatures [8]. When the outer protective cuticle is exposed to high temperatures, damage occurs in the form of splitting, cracking, or peeling of the cuticle resulting in acquired

Fig. 3.4 Straightened hair, styled with a barrel curling iron

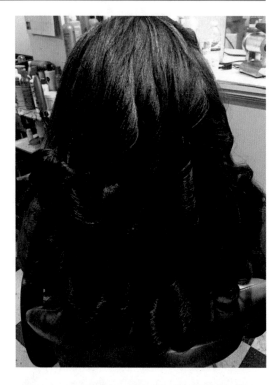

Fig. 3.5 Hooded blow-dryer

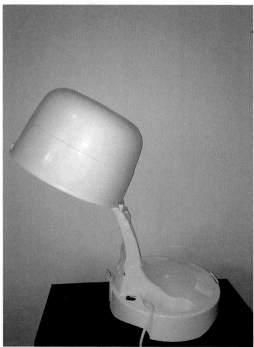

Fig. 3.6 The hair is wrapped circumferentially around the head before bedtime or after styling to maintain the underlying hairstyle

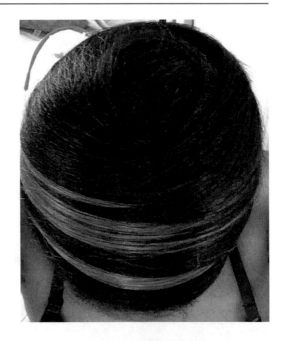

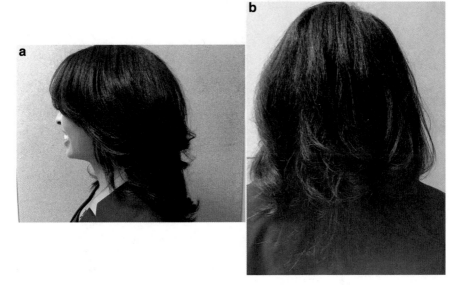

Fig. 3.7 (**a**, **b**) Blowout hairstyle

trichorrhexis nodosa and subsequent breakage [8–10]. Another common side effect of thermal straightening is the bubble hair defect, in which exposure of the hair shaft to elevated temperatures causes expulsion of water, in the form of vapor, out of the cortex and cuticle [3, 10, 11]. As a result, microscopic holes are left within the cuticle, which leaves the hair fragile and susceptible to breakage (Fig. 3.8) [3, 11].

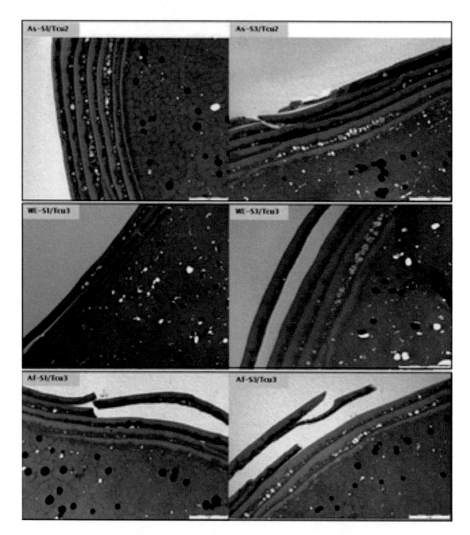

Fig. 3.8 Electron micrograph image of hair shafts following chemical straightening (*left column*) and a combination of chemical straightening and bleaching (*right column*) in Asian (*top row*) Caucasian (*middle row*) and African (*bottom row*) hair. In all hair types, holes can be appreciated within the cortex following chemical treatments, which is a sign of damage. Stripping of the top cuticular layers is also appreciated. (Reprinted from: Lee Y, Kim YD, Pi LQ, Lee SY, Hong H, Lee WS. Comparison of hair shaft damage after chemical treatment in Asian, White European, and African hair. Int J Dermatol. 2014 Sep;53(9):1103-10, with permission from John Wiley and Sons)

In addition to the previously described insults to the hair shaft, improper thermal straightening techniques can also cause local burns to the scalp, ears, and neck, which can result in infection and post-inflammatory dyspigmentation [5, 7].

Signs of thermal-induced damage may be observed on physical examination by the presence of broken hairs of varying lengths and splayed-apart distal hair shafts [9]. A tug test, which involves gently tugging the ends of a small number of hair fibers, will often result in the separation of small distal hair fragments [9]. Heat-induced damage is cumulative; therefore, frequent application of thermal styling tools causes progressive breakage and shortening of the hair [7, 8]. This damage is exacerbated when thermal straightening is applied to chemically treated hair [9].

Thermal straightening, specifically hot combing, has previously been implicated as a causative factor in scarring alopecia [12]. In 1968, LoPresti et al. described follicular scarring that was thought to be due to heated lubricating oils that drip down the hair shaft and burn the scalp, resulting in "hot comb alopecia" (see Chap. 10) [12]. Although scalp burns and hair shaft fragility have been directly linked to heat exposure, the association between hot combing and scarring alopecia has not been confirmed [5].

Prevention of Thermal Styling-Induced Hair Damage

It is important to assess the hair care and styling practices of all patients to identify sources of damage and breakage. Patients should be asked about the frequency of thermal styling, the tools used, and the temperature settings used [9]. Thermal straightening, especially hot combing should not be performed more than once a week and the temperature should not exceed 350 °F (or low/medium setting) [3, 9]. Although the use of hooded dryers significantly lengthens the drying and styling process, they provide a safer form of heat styling compared to handheld blow-dryers [8]. Hooded dryers diffuse evenly concentrated, lower intensity heat over a larger surface area and reduce breakage-inducing manipulation during the drying process [8]. Thermal styling should be further minimized on chemically straightened or dyed hair as it is less resistant to the insults of heat exposure. It is often beneficial to treat hair with a moisturizing deep conditioner or a heat protectant product prior to heat styling [8]. Heat protectants are often composed of silicones or other polymers that work by decreasing the transfer of heat to the hair shaft. However, it should be noted that despite best hair care practices, some hair textures will still be unable to withstand the stress of routine heat styling [8].

Brazilian Keratin Treatments/Formaldehyde-Based Straightening

Brazilian keratin straightening, also known as keratin smoothing or keratin straightening, is a newer method of hair straightening that has gained popularity as an alternative to chemical relaxers [13]. Based on manufacturer claims, these products claim to straighten the natural curl pattern of the hair, restore strength, and reduce "frizz," resulting in enhanced shine and manageability [14, 15]. While there are many different brands on the market, most keratin straightening treatments primarily consist of mixtures of hydrolyzed liquid keratin, formaldehyde solution, and conditioning cream [3, 13]. These treatments are typically recommended for salon use by certified specialists; however, newer products formulated for at-home use have recently been introduced into the commercial market [13].

During the process of keratin straightening, the hair is thoroughly washed and the formaldehyde/keratin solution is applied throughout the hair with a comb [3]. The hair is then blow-dried and flat ironed at elevated temperatures of 400–450 °F, which helps to seal the cuticle after straightening [13, 14]. The effects of these treatments typically last from 6 weeks to 5 months, depending on the specific product used and subsequent maintenance [13]. Many hairstylists suggest waiting 48–72 h before shampooing to allow the treatment to adequately set into the hair [13]. Because these chemicals are progressively removed from the hair with shampooing, most manufacturers and stylists recommend the use of "sulfate-free" shampoos or shampoos specifically formulated for keratin-treated hair to prolong the duration of results (see Chap. 7). This process is then repeated every few months, depending on the texture of the hair, and can be applied to previously treated hair. Unlike chemical relaxers, keratin straightening treatments are safe to use on color-treated hair [13].

This method of straightening differs from chemical relaxing in that the components do not permanently disrupt disulfide bonds, which is why this is considered a temporary straightening method [16]. During the initial washing phase of the keratin straightening process, exposure of the hair shaft to water results in disruption of hydrogen bonds within keratin molecules [16]. This temporarily resets the keratin into a straighter configuration, resulting in the more "loosened" curl pattern typically observed in wet hair [16]. This straightened keratin orientation is then maintained with the application of the hydrolyzed keratin and formaldehyde solution [13]. The formaldehyde (or its derivatives) acts as the cross-linking agents, which form bonds between the amino acids of the hydrolyzed liquid keratin and the hair's keratin molecules [13]. The cross-linked formaldehyde forms a hardened, water-resistant layer along the hair shafts, which maintains the straightened orientation of the hair for an extended period of time [3]. This reaction is enhanced by the application of heat, which helps seal the added keratin into the hair shaft [13]. The realigned and sealed keratin filaments provide enhanced shine and smoothness to the hair [16].

Hazards Associated with Brazilian Keratin Treatments

Since the introduction of Brazilian keratin straightening treatments, there have been growing concerns about the adverse effects of chronic formaldehyde exposure. Formaldehyde is a commonly used preservative and is used in the production of disinfectants, paints, pesticides, resins, and cosmetics [3, 17]. When heat is applied to formaldehyde-containing keratin treatments, formaldehyde gas is released, which has been associated with eye irritation, throat burning, and difficulty breathing [13].

There have also been concerns about the carcinogenic potential of chronic formaldehyde inhalation, which has been linked with an increased incidence of lymphohematopoietic malignancies [18, 19]. Current Occupational Safety and Health Administration (OSHA) guidelines indicate that manufacturers are required to disclose the presence of formaldehyde in their products and must include the words "potential cancer hazard" if the product is capable of releasing formaldehyde at levels above 0.5 ppm [17, 20]. OSHA regulations also require that salons adhere to worker safety guidelines, which include testing salon air during treatments to determine formaldehyde levels, providing adequate ventilation and protective equipment to employees performing treatments and training workers on the hazards of formaldehyde exposure [20].

These concerns have led to the development of "formaldehyde-free" keratin straightening products that contain glycolic acid or methylene glycol [3]. However, this labeling is misleading because these compounds degrade into formaldehyde when subjected to high temperatures [3]. This has led to the inclusion of methylene glycol-containing products in the OSHA safety guidelines regarding formaldehyde hair straightening products [20]. More recently, non-formaldehyde keratin straightening treatments, called "safe keratin treatments" (SKT), have been introduced into the market and contain hydrolyzed keratin, glyoxyloyl carbocysteine, glyoxyloyl keratin amino acids, silicone derivatives, and fatty acids [13, 14]. These products claim to provide similar straightening results compared to formaldehyde-containing keratin treatments. However, further research is needed to assess the relative safety and efficacy of these products [13].

References

1. Aryiku SA, Salam A, Dadzie OE, Jablonski NG. Clinical and anthropological perspectives on chemical relaxing of afro-textured hair. J Eur Acad Dermatol Venereol. 2015;29(9):1689–95.
2. Callender VD, McMichael AJ, Cohen GF. Medical and surgical therapies for alopecias in black women. Dermatol Ther. 2004;17(2):164–76.
3. Tanus A, Oliveira CC, Villarreal DJ, Sanchez FA, Dias MF. Black women's hair: the main scalp dermatoses and aesthetic practices in women of African ethnicity. An Bras Dermatol. 2015;90(4):450–65.
4. Bolduc C, Shapiro J. Hair care products: waving, straightening, conditioning, and coloring. Clin Dermatol. 2001;19(4):431–6.
5. McMichael AJ. Ethnic hair update: past and present. J Am Acad Dermatol. 2003;48(6 Suppl):S127–33.
6. Draelos ZD. Cosmetic dermatology: products and procedures. 1st ed. Chichester: Wiley-Blackwell; 2010.
7. Quinn CR, Quinn TM, Kelly AP. Hair care practices in African American women. Cutis. 2003;72(4):280–2, 285–9.
8. Davis-Sivasothy A. The science of black hair: a comprehensive guide to textured hair care. Stafford: Saja Publishing; 2011.
9. Mirmirani P. Ceramic flat irons: improper use leading to acquired trichorrhexis nodosa. J Am Acad Dermatol. 2010;62(1):145–7.
10. Roseborough IE, McMichael AJ. Hair care practices in African-American patients. Semin Cutan Med Surg. 2009;28(2):103–8.
11. Ruetsch SB, Kamath YK. Effects of thermal treatments with a curling iron on hair fiber. J Cosmet Sci. 2004;55(1):13–27.

12. LoPresti P, Papa CM, Kligman AM. Hot comb alopecia. Arch Dermatol. 1968;98(3):234–8.
13. Weathersby C, McMichael A. Brazilian keratin hair treatment: a review. J Cosmet Dermatol. 2013;12(2):144–8.
14. Keraluxe: how it works. 2016. Available from: https://kera-luxe.com/content/10-product-tutorial.
15. Keratin complex: the science. Available from: http://www.keratincomplex.com/about/the-science.
16. Gavazzoni Dias MF. Hair cosmetics: an overview. Int J Trichol. 2015;7(1):2–15.
17. Pierce JS, Abelmann A, Spicer LJ, Adams RE, Glynn ME, Neier K, et al. Characterization of formaldehyde exposure resulting from the use of four professional hair straightening products. J Occup Environ Hyg. 2011;8(11):686–99.
18. Beane Freeman LE, Blair A, Lubin JH, Stewart PA, Hayes RB, Hoover RN, et al. Mortality from lymphohematopoietic malignancies among workers in formaldehyde industries: the National Cancer Institute Cohort. J Natl Cancer Inst. 2009;101(10):751–61.
19. Hauptmann M, Lubin JH, Stewart PA, Hayes RB, Blair A. Mortality from lymphohematopoietic malignancies among workers in formaldehyde industries. J Natl Cancer Inst. 2003;95(21):1615–23.
20. United States Department of Labor, Occupational and Safety Health Administration (OSHA). Hair salons: facts about formaldehyde in hair products. 2012. Available from: https://www.osha.gov/SLTC/hairsalons/.

Ethnic Hairstyling Practices and Hair Prostheses I: Dreadlocks

4

Nashay N. Clemetson

Introduction

Popularized by the reggae icon Bob Marley, locks (also known as dreadlocks, locs, dreads, *ndiagne* [Senegal], *jatta* [Hindi]) have their roots in ancient traditions including African and Indian cultures, and religions including Rastafarianism and Hinduism [1, 2]. For many, the locking process is more than just a cosmetic endeavor, it is a spiritual experience. There are several different varieties of dreadlocks. "Freeform" locks vary in size, width, and length as the hair is allowed to become matted in a natural, untamed manner. "Salon" locks, such as sisterlocks and dreadlocks are preferred by many who desire a well-groomed appearance.

The overarching concept involves sectioning the hair into small locks that are then twisted, braided, or coiled using the fingers, palms, or special tools like a crochet hook or latch pin. The hair naturally mats over time with either approach [3]. Natural oils, such as coconut, olive, castor, and jojoba or commercially prepared pomades like beeswax are often added during styling. The locks are then groomed into elaborate styles or left to hang loosely. The new growth beneath the locked hair is twisted on average every 6–8 weeks, reintroducing tension of varying intensity (depending on the technique) on the roots [4]. For many, locks are a low-maintenance hairstyle mostly requiring shampooing the hair once or twice monthly and using natural oils for moisturizing 2–3 times per week.

Although there are many benefits of this increasingly popular hairstyling option, there are some undesirable sequelae to wearing dreadlocks. Locks that are improperly installed or maintained, retwisted and styled too tightly, or locks that are too long and heavy place the wearer at risk for irreversible alopecia (see Chap. 5).

N.N. Clemetson, M.D. (✉)
Department of Dermatology, The Johns Hopkins University School of Medicine, 5200 Eastern Avenue, MFL Center Tower Suite 2500, Baltimore, MD 21224, USA

© Springer International Publishing Switzerland 2017   43
C. Aguh, G.A. Okoye (eds.), *Fundamentals of Ethnic Hair*,
DOI 10.1007/978-3-319-45695-9_4

Lock Type

Any hair type will lock naturally, if left uncombed and unmanipulated for an extended period of time. There is no special guidance needed prior to this attempting this approach. Ideally, however, for the achievement of well-manicured locks, an individual should understand his or her hair type before locking of the hair is considered. The ability of the hair to lock and remained tightly intertwined depends on its structure (including curl pattern and fragility), growth rate, need for moisture/conditioning, and chemical alteration. Consultation with a natural hair specialist or dreadlocks specialist (loctician) is recommended prior to starting the locking process. This specialist can provide guidance in selecting the best locking technique based on hair type and maintaining the health of the scalp and locks. They can also help the individual decide whether the "big chop" (see Chap. 8) or using temporary extensions before starting the locking process is beneficial.

Dreadlocks

The word "dread" was initially used to describe the fear invoked by the appearance of the knotted and matted hairs worn by members of the Rastafarian movement. It was believed that the wearing of dreadlocks symbolized the individual's dismissal of the importance of vanity and beauty. These thick, long, tightly locks flow freely off the scalp and can come to rest as far down as the ankles, depending on the individual (Fig. 4.1). The formation of dreadlocks involves several techniques that will be discussed later in this chapter.

Sisterlocks

Created and trademarked in 1993 by Dr. JoAnne Cornwell, an associate professor of Africana Studies and French at San Diego University, sisterlocks were designed for women of African heritage. The locks are created using a special looped pin trademarked by the company. Their installation and maintenance are done by specialists trained and licensed in this technique. The parting of the hair and the tool used vary depending on the hair type and texture. No hair products are required with this technique. The locks consist of a few strands of hair and are very thin, increasing their susceptibility to breakage (Fig. 4.2a, b). The thin strands often appear unbraided and unlocked, facilitating the wearing of styles that thicker, bulkier locks do not. When worn by men, they are called "brotherlocks".

Lock Formation

Traditionally, it was believed that in order to create locks, an individual had to refrain from brushing, combing, or cutting the hair. This method created locks that varied greatly in size, width, shape, length, and texture. The method has come to be

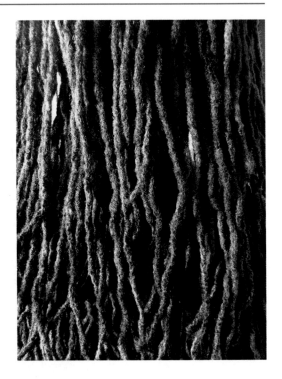

Fig. 4.1 Close-up of dreadlocks

known as the "neglect" method. Other names for this method include "organic" or "patience" methods. Similarly, "freeform" locks are created by allowing the hair to knit together naturally into locks of varying sizes. Freeform locks are patterned to a degree, as the hair is separated in "chunks" (not parted as with a comb) into fairly determinate sections after washing.

Once the locking technique is chosen, the hair is prepped for initiation. Ideally, at least 3 in. of new growth (hair that has not been chemically processed) is needed. Some individuals with chemically processed hair may choose not to cut the processed strands in order to maintain the hair length. They should be advised that this portion of the hair may not lock. The hair is washed with an acidic shampoo and then rinsed. This is repeated until the hair and scalp are clean. An apple cider vinegar rinse, moisturizing conditioner, or hot oil treatment may then be used. The hair is then partially dried using low heat or blotted with a towel.

Starting at the nape of the neck, the hair is sectioned into small polygonal areas, often squares or triangles. The size of the section determines the thickness of the lock. For thicker and fewer locks, the area is made larger. For thinner and fuller-appearing locks, the area is made smaller. For individuals with thinner or less dense hair, fewer locks are ideal. There is less tension therefore less susceptibility to hair breakage, lock thinning, and alopecia when each individual lock has more volume.

Fig. 4.2 (**a, b**) Sisterlocks

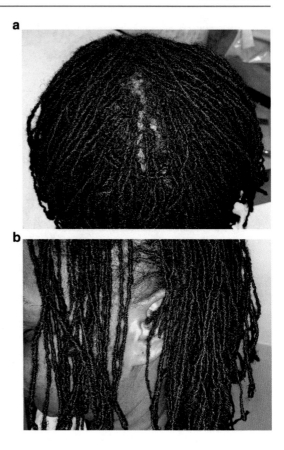

Several products, depending on individual/stylist preference, hair type, and lock technique, may then be used as the locking process begins. Products include permanent bonding agents (like glues), protein gels, commercially prepared locking pomades, waxes and creams, and natural oils and butters [5]. The use of bonding agents is discouraged; they increase the risk of breakage, scalp inflammation, and hair loss. Protein gels, while they harden the hair, do not allow the hair to move freely and twist on itself. The locking process is therefore slower. There is a wide variety of commercially prepared pomades and waxes. They contain ingredients that provide various degrees of hold, while adding sheen and pleasant fragrances. A major drawback of pomades, waxes, and creams is the accumulation of buildup within the locks [5]. Removal of buildup can be difficult, and in some case may require cutting of the locks. Using natural oils that are liquid at room temperature results in well-moisturized locks with less buildup.

Palm Rolling

Palm rolling is the most common technique used in locking hair. It is very simple and requires minimal technical skills. After applying a thin layer of products (wax, gel, or oil), the loose hair or new growth around the roots is separated from nearby sections/locks and wrapped around the lock. The lock is then rolled clockwise between the base of the palms, starting from the root, and gradually descending the shaft to the ends. With each 360° roll, the lock is temporarily released and then rolled again. This requires applying significant tension and twisting forces to the hair and scalp. This technique can be used to start locks or retwist mature locks. Palm rolling compresses and tightens new growth into existing locks. This maintains uniformity in size and smoothens the locks. The process is repeated every 6–8 weeks, especially after the hair is washed, as the immature portion of the lock will unravel.

Interlocking

Interlocking is the quickest method to create instant locks and also a great lock maintenance technique. The sectioned hair is twisted or braided on the ends and the new growth is separated from neighboring locks and wrapped around the base of the respective lock. The lock is then crocheted using a latch pin (tool that hooks the lock and loops it through on itself) or a crochet needle in alternating directions (north–south, east–west, and diagonally) (Fig. 4.3a–c).

The looping or folding, however, creates unnatural twisting of the hair strands, producing tension and increased susceptibility to breakage. The tools also rip hairs within the locks causing micro-tears that over time weaken and thin the lock. When retwisting at the roots, the constant pulling also creates micro-fractures near the scalp, and over time the entire lock may loosen and break. Adding to the trauma of this process, styling of interlocked locks prolongs the tension on the scalp, worsening hair breakage and loss. Interlocked hair may be washed immediately as it does not unravel. When repeated every 3–6 months and done by locticians who are well trained in this technique, the adverse risks of using this technique are reduced.

Backcombing

Unlike the previously mentioned techniques, which can be used to maintain already formed locks, backcombing can be used to initiate dreadlocks and does not require a big chop. This method may be preferable for individuals with straight hair at least 6 in. long, such as people of Caucasian and Asian descent, and people of African descent who have chemically relaxed hair.

It is a teasing of the strands to give a "ratted" look. When used in the locking process, the section of hair chosen for the lock is held firmly at the ends of the

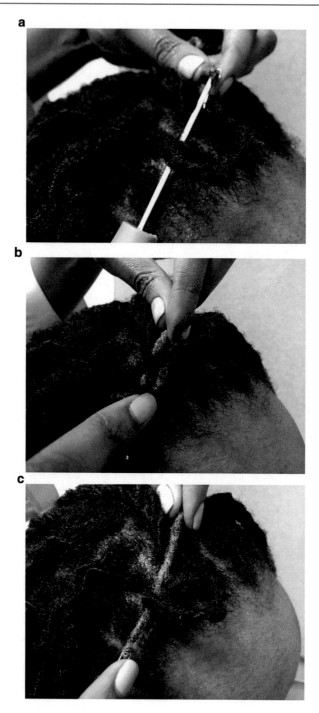

Fig. 4.3 (a–c) Interlocking technique

hair. Using a fine-toothed comb in the dominant hand, the hair is pushed down-ward from about 3 in. above the scalp, toward the scalp. The hand holding the section rotates between 0 and 180° and the strand is twirled constantly while the comb moves down the shaft. There should be an even fuzz ball at the root when the comb is removed. The hair should be packed tightly against the forming locks with each stroke of the comb. Loose strands on the shaft are acceptable. A rubber band may be applied to the end of the lock to reduce the chances of frizz-ing or fraying. The lock may then be gently rolled in the palms, using light moisturizers or oils. As the lock matures over several months, they assume a matted appearance (Fig. 4.4). The locks are then maintained using palm rolling or other techniques.

Freeform

Freeform locks are ideal for anyone who prefers the least hands-on lock main-tenance. The hair is washed and then allowed to mat and lock naturally over weeks to months (Fig. 4.5). Matting occurs quickly, but the hair appears ung-roomed compared to other type of locks, and may be less cosmetically

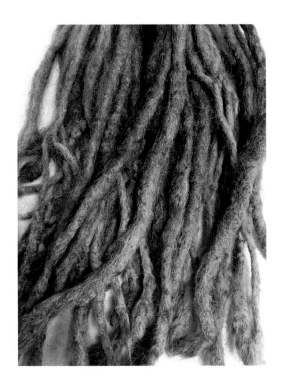

Fig. 4.4 Recently shorn dreadlocks, created using the "backcombing" technique

Fig. 4.5 Freeform
dreadlocks in a Rastafarian
man

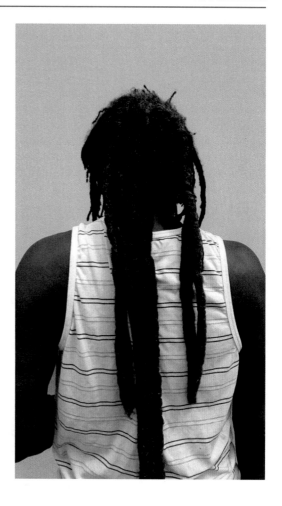

appealing to some. The locks vary in size, length, and bulk. There is no manipulation of the hair except when washed. Depending on the individual, natural oils
may be applied to the scalp and hair. The roots may be brushed and the locks
wrapped to give a neat appearance, especially for professionals and special
events. This is the most economical and least time-consuming technique.

Lock Maintenance

The maintenance of locks parallels other natural hair care recommendations.
Like other natural hairstyles, locks should be washed and conditioned regularly.
For those with excessive dryness, hot-oil or deep conditioning treatments every
4–6 weeks are ideal. Retwisting/tightening may be done as often as weekly (for

palm-rolled locks) to never (for freeform locks). It is important to choose locticians/natural hair stylists carefully, since people untrained in lock techniques may employ unsafe practices that lead to temporary or permanent alopecia.

After washing and conditioning, the hair should be thoroughly dried, in order to prevent the growth of mold in the warm moist locks. Lightly brushing the hair is acceptable but combing is discouraged. If the hair is permanently dyed, extra moisturization is needed to prevent dryness and decreased fragility.

Conclusion

Locking offers individuals of all ethnic and racial backgrounds a stylish, affordable, and hassle-free option of wearing their hair in an unprocessed, natural state. There are a variety of locking techniques that can be used to start and maintain this hairstyle, offering freedom of expression and individuality. The choice to wear locks is a personal one and it may be spiritually and/or politically motivated. It is in the dermatologist's best interest, as he/she cares for patients, to be able to offer guidance on hair and scalp health and the benefits and risks of these hairstyles.

References

1. Persadsingh N. The hair in black women. Kingston: N. Persadsingh; 2003.
2. Mastalia F, Pagano A. Dreads. New York: Artisan; 1999.
3. Khumalo NP. African skin and hair disorders, an issue of dermatologic clinics. London: Elsevier Health Sciences; 2014.
4. Gathers RC, Jankowski M, Eide M, Lim HW. Hair grooming practices and central centrifugal cicatricial alopecia. J Am Acad Dermatol. 2009;60(4):574–8.
5. Reed-Johnson M. The world of dreadlocks: beyond maturity. Victoria: Trafford; 2005.

Ethnic Hairstyling Practices and Hair Prostheses II: Wigs, Weaves, and Other Extensions

5

Alessandra Haskin and Crystal Aguh

Introduction

Hairstyles vary significantly across ethnic populations and are often thought of as an expression of personal style and a celebration of cultural heritage. This chapter provides an overview of the wide variety of hairstyles and hair prostheses most commonly used in the black community as well as the potential harmful effects associated with them. It also includes a brief discussion of camouflage techniques for patients with hair loss.

Ethnic Hairstyling Practices and Hair Prostheses

Braids and Twists

Braids and twists, created with or without extensions, are popular hairstyles in women of African descent and offer a relatively low maintenance, chemical-free method of hairstyling [1]. Hair braiding, or hair plaiting, can be accomplished by interlocking three pieces of hair together in sections, which can extend from the scalp at varying lengths (Fig. 5.1). Microbraids are very small braids, typically 2–4mm in diameter, which are created using the same process. "Cornrows" are another type of braid in which three pieces of hair are interlocked and laid flat along

A. Haskin, B.A.
Howard University College of Medicine, 520 W St. NW, Washington, DC 20059, USA

C. Aguh, M.D. (✉)
Department of Dermatology, Johns Hopkins University School of Medicine,
5200 Eastern Avenue, Suite 2500, Baltimore, MD 21224, USA

© Springer International Publishing Switzerland 2017
C. Aguh, G.A. Okoye (eds.), *Fundamentals of Ethnic Hair*,
DOI 10.1007/978-3-319-45695-9_5

Fig. 5.1 Braids or plaits. These are created by sectioning the hair and interlocking three pieces of hair. These can be done with the individual's hair or with the addition of extensions

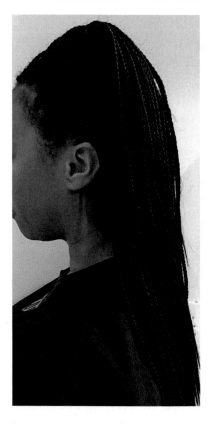

the scalp in stationary rows/lines or geometric designs (Fig. 5.2). Twists are created by dividing small pieces of hair into two sections and wrapping them around each other (Fig. 5.3). These braided or twisted styles are held together using styling gel or beeswax and may last up to several weeks [1, 2]. Pieces of human or synthetic hair fibers, often referred to as extensions, can be added to any one of these styles by braiding/twisting them in with the natural hair to increase volume and length (Fig. 5.4) [1].

Weaves and Extensions

The use of hair weaves and extensions has become a popular styling practice for many ethnic groups [3]. These hair prostheses are used to add volume and length to existing hair and can be applied using many different techniques. Human hair weaves are most commonly obtained internationally from Asian women who grow and sell their hair for commercial use [4]. The hair is then processed with dyes and chemical waving products to alter the hair into a variety of colors and textures to mimic the appearance of the customer's hair (Fig. 5.5) [4]. The use of human hair extensions provides the versatility of one's own hair, in that it can be modified with

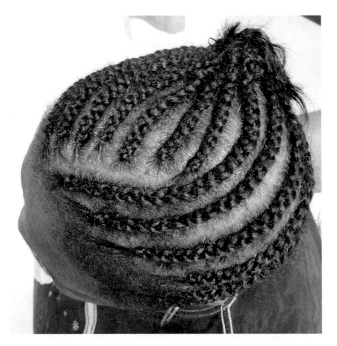

Fig. 5.2 Cornrows. A type of braid in which three pieces of hair are interlocked and laid flat along the scalp in stationary rows/lines or geometric designs. These can be done with the individual's hair or with the addition of extensions

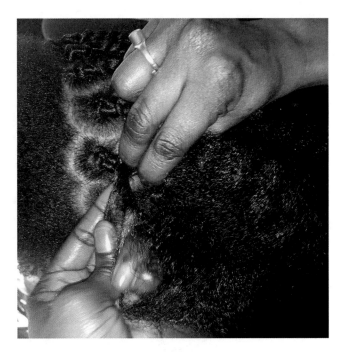

Fig. 5.3 Twists are created by dividing small pieces of hair into two sections and wrapping them around each other

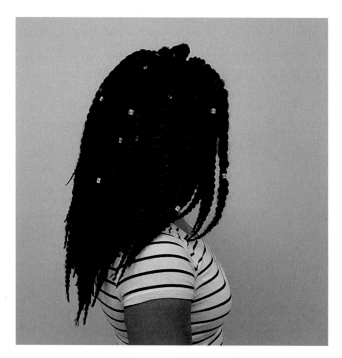

Fig. 5.4 Extension are pieces of human or synthetic hair fibers that can be braided or twisted in with the natural hair to increase volume and length

Fig. 5.5 Human hair used for hair weaves are processed with dyes and chemical waving products to create a variety of colors and textures

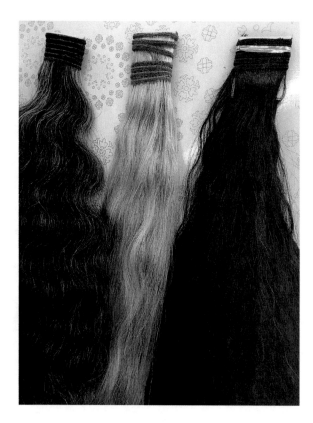

traditional styling tools [5]. Synthetic hair weaves are composed of modacrylic which is formed from two polymerized monomers, acrylonitrile and vinyl chloride [4, 6]. These fibers are heated and strung into strands of varying diameters, curl patterns, and colors to match the appearance of natural hair shafts [6]. However, the styling of synthetic hair fibers is permanent and cannot be altered with thermal styling tools since these fibers melt when exposed to high temperatures.

One of the most popular methods of hair weave application involves the use of extensions called "hair tracts", which are created using machines that sew small pieces of hair together onto a tract (Fig. 5.6). The individual's hair is braided into cornrows and the extensions are sewn onto the cornrows with needle and thread (Fig. 5.7) [1]. Weaving nets can also be used to attach hair extensions and are particularly useful in patients suffering from hair loss. A thin, netted material is laid on top of a section of cornrows and attached to the perimeter of the braided portion of the head. The extensions are then sewn directly onto the net, instead of the cornrows, which can relieve some of the tension applied to the patient's underlying hair. Hair extensions can also be applied with the use of clips or tape, which attach to the patient's existing hair [5].

Alternatively, individual hair fibers or hair tracts can be applied using adhesives such as latex-based bonding glues [3]. The latter can be applied by lining the tract of the hair extensions with bonding glue and affixing it to the base of the hair shaft [3]. These glued-in hair extensions can then be removed with specially designed solvents [6]. Removal of glued-on hair extensions can often result in significant hair breakage. The solvents used for removal can also cause scalp irritation and irritant contact dermatitis [6]. Bonding glue can also be used to fuse individual human or synthetic hair fibers to the base of natural hair shafts

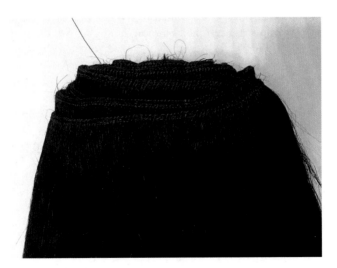

Fig. 5.6 Extensions ("hair tracts") are created using machines that sew small pieces of hair together onto a strip (tracts)

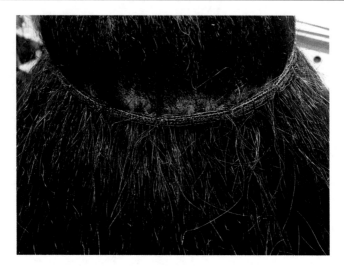

Fig. 5.7 In sewn-in hair weaves, the individual's hair is braided into cornrows and the hair tracts are sewn onto the cornrows with needle and thread

using a glue gun [5, 6]. These bonded hair extensions typically remain in place for up to 8 weeks but may loosen or fall out sooner in individuals with excessive sebum production [5, 6]. Bonded extensions are removed by melting the glue with the tip of a glue gun, pulling out the added hair pieces, and removing excess glue with the application of peanut oil [6]. Many of the adhesive agents used in both types of bonding glues contain latex and polyacrylates, which have been associated with the development of allergic contact dermatitis [5–8]. These hair attachment techniques can result in unavoidable hair breakage and scalp burns and are therefore not recommended [6]. When properly applied, sewn-in hair extensions are the preferred method of attaching hair to the scalp.

Wigs

Wigs are scalp prostheses that are temporarily affixed to the scalp to cover the underlying hair. While wigs can be made using various techniques, one of the most common methods involves knotting or sewing small pieces of human or synthetic hair to a foundation made of netting, silk, or similar materials (Fig. 5.8) [5]. Prior to donning a wig, the underlying hair is firmly held flat against the scalp with the use of a wig cap, usually made of cotton, nylon, or satin (Fig. 5.9). The wig is then attached using materials such as combs, clips, tapes, or bonding glue (Fig. 5.10). More recently, some wigs are created using a polyurethane base, which more closely resembles the human scalp, and pieces of hair are inserted into this base for a more natural look [5]. Lacefront wigs are also quite popular as they contain a transparent attachment that allows for more realistic simulation of the frontal hairline (Fig. 5.11).

Fig. 5.8 Small pieces of human or synthetic hair are knotted or sewn onto a foundation made of netting, silk, or similar materials

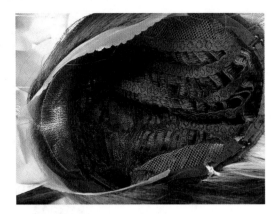

Fig. 5.9 Wigs are attached using materials such as combs, clips, tapes, or bonding glue

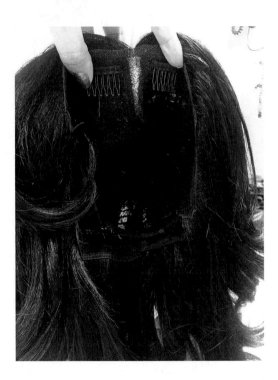

Unlike other types of extensions, wigs do not require the presence of underlying hair. They are therefore a popular styling options for women hoping to conceal moderate to severe hair loss. This is particularly useful for women who are undergoing chemotherapy during cancer treatments (Table 5.1). Table 5.2 provides detailed descriptions of common types of wigs and hairpieces.

Fig. 5.10 Prior to donning a wig, the underlying hair is firmly held flat against the scalp with the use of a wig cap, usually made of cotton, nylon, or satin

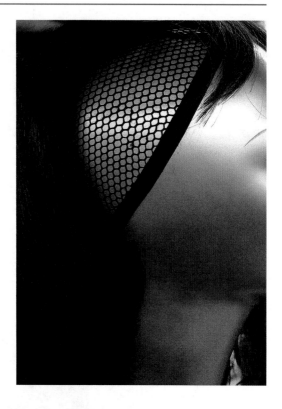

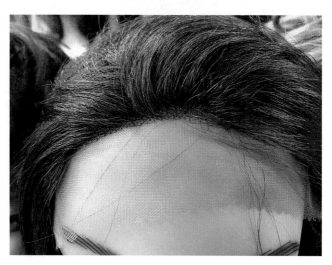

Fig. 5.11 Lacefront wigs contain a transparent attachment that allows for more realistic simulation of the frontal hairline

Table 5.1 Patient perspective

I sat there, newly diagnosed with *moderately differentiated invasive ductal carcinoma* in my right breast, beginning chemotherapy in two weeks. I was not surprised that hair loss is associated with chemotherapy treatment. However being quite frank, I was more concerned with the side effects: nausea, lethargy, weight loss, compromised immune system, neuropathy, constipation, etc. Knowing that I would be losing my hair spoke to my vanity

I've worn u-part wigs, full sew-in wigs, clip-ins, in the past but after my diagnosis I decided I'd be graduating to lace front wigs. I'd need to have it custom made and colored

It has been two months, and unfortunately, I am not excited about this wig. The lace color does not match my skin tone, nor does it cover in front of my ears very well. So I ended up looking like I have a well styled mop on my head. Thankfully, I can manipulate it well enough, but I still will be getting a new wig made

Truth be told, there are restrictions that make wearing a lace front wig (or any wig for that matter) difficult for cancer patients. I cannot wear glue to secure the lace front wig because my skin is too sensitive. I've had chemical burns on my face from my usual acne facial washes. The fit for wigs can be too tight for some patients. I've been able to stretch the wig, making it comfortable. That took a few attempts

At this point, I'm happy that I have a wig so I can look normal. I wear make-up to cover the blotchy discolorations on my face, and I manage chemotherapy side effects as gracefully as I can. Most days are great days. I am not keen on being stared at with a bald head, so I wear my wig daily. I couldn't imagine leaving home without it. Some ladies would object strongly to my regular use of my wig, but to each their own. I like looking normal, with my wig

Table 5.2 Descriptions of wig types

Type of wig	Description	Comments
• Wefted wigs	• Consist of a cap with machine-wefted rows of synthetic hair	• Inexpensive • Often have a less natural look • Very durable
• Monofilament wigs	• Consist of a fine lace material known as "monofilament," in which hair fibers are individually knotted to the lace	• Can be expensive • Allow the hair to be brushed and parted in any direction, providing a more natural look
• Lace front wigs	• A thin piece of lace, extending from ear to ear, is attached to the front of a wig. The lace is glued to the forehead	• Gives the appearance of natural hair growth at the frontal hairline
• Integration wigs	• A special type of wig cap designed to allow the patient's natural hair to be pulled through openings in the wig	• Can provide a more natural look by allowing the patient's hair to be blended with the wig hair
• Partial coverage wigs/hairpieces	• *Toupee*: circular hairpiece frequently used to cover male-pattern hair loss.	• Ideal for coverage of localized areas of hair loss
	• *Wiglet*: Small hair pieces that can be used to add bangs to the anterior scalp or fullness to the top of the scalp	• All forms can be attached to the scalp using clips or adhesive tapes
	• *¾ Cap Wig:* smaller wigs designed to cover most of the scalp, except for the frontal and temporal hairlines	

(continued)

Table 5.2 (continued)

Type of wig	Description	Comments
• Custom-made wigs	• Developed to ensure a precise fit and involves making a plaster mold of the patient's scalp and manufacturing a silicone or polyurethane vacuum-based wig	• Very expensive and can take up to 6 months to acquire
	• Requires that the patient maintain a bald scalp	• Can cost between $1000 and $2000
	• Air is expelled as the wigs is progressively pushed down on the scalp creating a tight seal	• Require same type of grooming as human hair

Hair Damage Associated with Hairstyling Practices

While many of the previously described hairstyling practices often improve the manageability of ethnic hair and promote ease of everyday styling, improper use can result in hair loss.

Traction Alopecia

Traction alopecia (TA) is a condition characterized by hair loss along the frontal hairline and occurs as a direct result of hairstyles that apply excess tension to the frontal scalp (Fig. 5.12). This has become a growing problem in patients who continually wear hair weaves and extensions [4]. Many of these hairstyles add extra weight to the hair and can result in severe breakage due to increased tension applied to a small number of hair shafts [9]. The application of excessively tight braids and/or weaves can often result in pain and the formation of "pimples" over the follicles with greatest tension, which are symptoms that have been linked to the development of TA [10]. The highest prevalence of TA has been reported in patients who combine hairstyling practices; specifically, the application of tension in the form of weaves, braids, and twists (with or without hair extensions) to chemically treated hair [10–12]. Dreadlocks are also associated with a high likelihood of developing traction alopecia. Similarly, thermal straightening can lead to weakening of the hair shaft, resulting in additional breakage when traction is applied [13].

Scarring Alopecia

Studies have shown that the use of hair weaves, cornrows, and braided hairstyles is more prevalent among women who develop central centrifugal cicatricial alopecia (CCCA) (see Chap. 10) [14]. The authors believe that patients with CCCA should be discouraged from wearing hairstyles that may increase tension or add

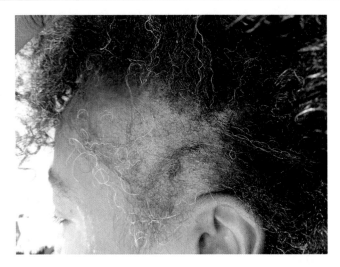

Fig. 5.12   Traction alopecia

weight to the hair along the scalp vertex, particularly long heavy dreadlocks or tightly braided extensions. However, the specific role of these hairstyling practices in the development of CCCA is yet to be confirmed. In these cases, the use of wigs or weaves sewn over a net may be preferable to avoid further trauma to the vertex scalp.

Scalp Infections

The presence of braids and weaves can make it difficult to thoroughly cleanse the hair, resulting in a higher incidence of seborrheic dermatitis, bacterial folliculitis, and fungal infections of the scalp [2, 3]. A higher incidence of carrier-state tinea capitis has been reported in African American women, and hairstyling practices have been postulated to be contributing factors. The frequent use of traction-inducing hairstyles and subsequent hair shaft damage may provide easier access to fungal penetration. Additionally low frequency of shampooing may lead to inadequate fungal spore removal [15].

Recommendations for Installing and Wearing Extensions

Patients may be reluctant to remove braided styles and hair weaves because obtaining these hairstyles can often be expensive and time consuming. It is important that patients be educated about the potential deleterious effects of these hairstyling practices, including indicators of scalp inflammation and hair shaft damage such as pain, pimples, stinging, or crusting [16]. Ideally, braided styles and hair weaves should be worn for limited periods of time, with breaks of a few weeks between hairstyles, to allow the

Fig. 5.13 Allergic contact dermatitis caused by the chemicals used in the processing of human and synthetic hair weaves

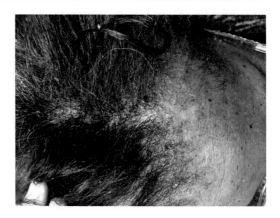

Table 5.3 Hairstyling recommendations

- Loosen the application of braids, especially around the hairline
- Leave braided styles in the hair for no longer than 2–3 months
- Opt for larger diameter braids and dreadlocks
- Hair extensions should only be used sparingly for short periods of time and immediately removed if they are causing pain or irritation
- When applying weaves, avoid using bonding glues; instead, opt for loosely sewn-in weaves
- Remove hair weaves/extensions every 3–4 weeks
- Take extra care to thoroughly cleanse the scalp, especially areas that are difficult to access due to the presence of braids and/or hair weaves
- Take breaks between wearing braided and/or sewn-in styles
- Extra caution should be used when manipulating chemically treated hair
- When possible, give hair a break from all styling practices to allow it to recover from stress. This can be done by adopting a natural hairstyle or by temporarily protecting the hair with the use of wigs or scarfs

hair to recover from prolonged tension [6]. Also, the chemicals used in the processing of human and synthetic hair weaves can induce an allergic contact dermatitis (Fig. 5.13). Therefore, patients are advised to wash hair weaves prior to installation. Table 5.3 outlines general hairstyling recommendations that can be used to help patients stop the progression of or prevent hair loss caused by these hairstyling practices.

The use of wigs can be an easy way to cover and protect the hair by decreasing the amount of physical trauma; however, they can also induce damage to the underlying hair. Clips and adhesives applied to the hairline can cause breakage, especially with repeated use [5]. Adhesive tapes and bonds can also induce allergic and irritant contact dermatitis [5]. Cotton and nylon wig caps can also cause hair loss due to constant friction at the hairline, which can weaken the hair shaft. It is not uncommon to find patients suffering from one form of hair loss to develop a secondary traction alopecia from the repeated use of tightly fitted wig caps [12]. This material also absorbs moisture and can leave the hair dry and even more susceptible to breakage. Therefore, the use of satin or silk wig caps is preferred.

Considerations for Camouflaging Hair Loss

Alopecia is a common problem among men and women and can be a significantly distressing experience. Many patients come to their dermatologist to seek guidance and advice about ways to hide or decrease the appearance of hair loss. Therefore, it is important to have suggestions or resources for these patients. In addition to some of the hairstyling methods previously discussed in this chapter, there are also other techniques that can be used to camouflage hair loss. Patients may initially present with concerns about "thinning" hair, especially if the scalp is visible [17]. Scalp visibility can have a significant negative impact on quality of life in patients with alopecia [18]. Scalp camouflaging agents such as hair filler fibers, scalp sprays, and hair crayons can be used for this purpose [17]. These agents reduce the appearance of the scalp by decreasing the color contrast between the patient's hair and scalp skin and provide an illusion of increased hair density [17].

One of the most popular products used to camouflage the scalp is topical hair filler fibers. These products consist of wool keratin particles that are positively charged and cling to the negatively charged terminal and vellus hairs of the scalp via electrostatic forces [17]. They are applied by sprinkling the fibers on the affected area of the scalp daily, which can be followed with the application of hairspray to facilitate increased binding of the fibers to the patient's scalp [17]. These products are not effective for patients with complete or significant hair loss as there must be existing hair for the filler fibers to bind to [17]. Camouflaging lotions, sprays, and hair crayons work similarly by depositing color on the hair and scalp, creating the appearance of increased density of hair follicles. These products are frequently used in conjunction with topical medications for hair loss and are safe to use following hair transplantation [17]. It is important to note that when these products are used concurrently with topical minoxidil, the minoxidil should be applied first and allowed to dry before adding the camouflaging agents [17]. These agents should also be removed before the next application of minoxidil [17]. Scalp tattooing has become popular as a permanent camouflage option and is especially useful for patients with bitemporal hair loss or miniaturization [6]. Small dots are tattooed on the scalp to resemble hair follicles and create the illusion of more fullness at the anterior hairline [6, 17].

Patients should choose a camouflage technique that works best for their pattern and extent of hair loss. However, it is important that these styles do not compromise the application of necessary medical therapies, such as topical or intralesional steroids and minoxidil. Patients should be reminded that wigs and hairpieces that can be easily removed are preferred while undergoing treatment. Weaves or other hairstyles that limit accessibility to the scalp decrease the ability to apply at home treatments. They also hinder a thorough scalp examination and should therefore be removed prior to their dermatology appointments.

References

1. Callender VD, McMichael AJ, Cohen GF. Medical and surgical therapies for alopecias in black women. Dermatol Ther. 2004;17(2):164–76.

2. Quinn CR, Quinn TM, Kelly AP. Hair care practices in African American women. Cutis. 2003;72(4):280–2, 285–9.
3. Roseborough IE, McMichael AJ. Hair care practices in African-American patients. Semin Cutan Med Surg. 2009;28(2):103–8.
4. Draelos ZD. Cosmetics: an overview. Curr Probl Dermatol. 1995;7(2):45–64.
5. Banka N, Bunagan MJ, Dubrule Y, Shapiro J. Wigs and hairpieces: evaluating dermatologic issues. Dermatol Ther. 2012;25(3):260–6.
6. Draelos ZD. Hair care: an illustrated dermatologic handbook. London: Taylor & Francis; 2005.
7. Mimura T. Bilateral eyelid erythema associated with false eyelash glue. Cutan Ocul Toxicol. 2013;32(1):89–90.
8. Weber-Muller F, Reichert-Penetrat S, Schmutz JL, Barbaud A. Contact dermatitis from poly-acrylate in TENS electrode. Ann Dermatol Venereol. 2004;131(5):478–80.
9. McMichael AJ. Ethnic hair update: past and present. J Am Acad Dermatol. 2003;48(6 Suppl):S127–33.
10. Khumalo NP, Jessop S, Gumedze F, Ehrlich R. Determinants of marginal traction alopecia in African girls and women. J Am Acad Dermatol. 2008;59(3):432–8.
11. Khumalo NP, Jessop S, Gumedze F, Ehrlich R. Hairdressing and the prevalence of scalp disease in African adults. Br J Dermatol. 2007;157(5):981–8.
12. Haskin A, Aguh C. All hairstyles are not created equal: what the dermatologist needs to know about black hairstyling practices and the risk of traction alopecia (TA). J Am Acad Dermatol. 2016;75:606–11.
13. Semble AL, McMichael AJ. Hair loss in patients with skin of color. Semin Cutan Med Surg. 2015;34(2):81–8.
14. Gathers RC, Lim HW. Central centrifugal cicatricial alopecia: past, present, and future. J Am Acad Dermatol. 2009;60(4):660–8.
15. Silverberg NB, Weinberg JM, DeLeo VA. Tinea capitis: focus on African American women. J Am Acad Dermatol. 2002;46(2 Suppl Understanding):S120–4.
16. Mirmirani P, Khumalo NP. Traction alopecia: how to translate study data for public education—closing the KAP gap? Dermatol Clin. 2014;32(2):153–61.
17. Donovan JC, Shapiro RL, Shapiro P, Zupan M, Pierre-Louis M, Hordinsky MK. A review of scalp camouflaging agents and prostheses for individuals with hair loss. Dermatol Online J. 2012;18(8):1.
18. Dlova NC, Fabbrocini G, Lauro C, Spano M, Tosti A, Hift RH. Quality of life in South African Black women with alopecia: a pilot study. Int J Dermatol. 2015;55:875–81.

Ethnic Hair Care Products

6

Alessandra Haskin and Crystal Aguh

Introduction

The multibillion dollar market for black hair care and styling products is constantly growing and changing [1]. These products are tailored to satisfy the unique hair care needs of black consumers (and others with curly hair) and are often located in a separate section of the cosmetics aisle in retail stores and pharmacies. This section will discuss the use of hair oils, butters, and various styling aids commonly used by those with tightly curled hair [2]. It is important that dermatologists become aware of these frequently used hair care and styling aids, and understand how they affect the hair.

Hair Oils

Oils have been a vital component of black hair care for centuries and are frequently included in a vast number of hair care products [3]. Although there have been a limited number of studies and published data about the effects of oils on the hair and skin, generations of women have observed the importance of oils for moisture retention, hair growth, and protection from damage.

A. Haskin, B.A.
Howard University College of Medicine, 520 W St. NW, Washington, DC 20059, USA

C. Aguh, M.D. (✉)
Department of Dermatology, Johns Hopkins University School of Medicine,
5200 Eastern Avenue, Suite 2500, Baltimore, MD 21224, USA

© Springer International Publishing Switzerland 2017   67
C. Aguh, G.A. Okoye (eds.), *Fundamentals of Ethnic Hair*,
DOI 10.1007/978-3-319-45695-9_6

Synthetic Hair Oils

Petroleum-based oils such as petrolatum and mineral oil (liquid petroleum) have traditionally been the most commonly used oils in black hair care [3]. These oils are often the primary ingredients in solid emollients, often referred to as pomades or "hair grease." These products typically contain mixtures of petrolatum, mineral oil, vegetable oil, and lanolin and are used for various purposes such as hair and scalp lubrication and protection during thermal and chemical straightening [4]. These ingredients can also be formulated into aerosolized products, commonly referred to as "oil sheen sprays," which are typically used as finishing aids to add luster and shine [5]. In addition to its large molecular size, mineral oil is a hydrocarbon and therefore has no affinity for hair proteins [6]. Thus, despite the improved manageability and softness that petroleum-based oils provide, they do not penetrate into the hair shaft [3]. Instead, these oils coat the surface of the cuticle and are effective at preventing moisture loss from the hair shaft [3]. Another benefit of mineral oil is its ability to spread evenly on the hair surface, which helps to decrease damage during combing and reduces split end formation [7]. Some patients will resort to heavy application of these products to the scalp in hopes of masking underlying scalp conditions such as seborrheic dermatitis, when in fact it may actually exacerbate this condition [2].

Natural Hair Oils: Essential Oils

Essential oils are plant-based oils that are commonly used in hair care for their sensory effects on the scalp and their medicinal properties [3]. Some examples include rosemary, peppermint, tea tree, cedarwood, lavender, thyme, and ylang ylang essential oils [3]. Many of these oils function as scalp stimulants and are used to soothe dryness and irritation [3]. Specifically, rosemary oil has been reported to promote hair growth and has antifungal properties that can help address conditions like seborrheic dermatitis [8, 9]. A small number of studies have also reported on the specific anti-inflammatory and hair growth promoting effects of *Zizyphus jujuba* essential oil, also known as jujube oil [10, 11]. However, essential oils are extremely potent and can cause redness, burning, and irritation when applied to the scalp alone. Therefore, they must be diluted with carrier oils before being applied to the skin or hair [12]. When massaged into the scalp, mixtures of essential oils and carrier oils have been shown to stimulate hair growth in alopecia areata (Table 6.1) [13]. It is important to note that all patients, especially those who are pregnant or nursing or have other medical conditions such as hypertension or epilepsy, should not use certain essential oils such as thyme oil. Please consult with your healthcare provider prior to using any essential oils.

Table 6.1 Sample oil mixture for treatment of alopecia areata

3 drops of lavender oil
2 drops of thyme oil
2 drops of cedarwood oil
2 drops of rosemary oil
3 mL of jojoba oil
20 mL of grapeseed oil

Natural Hair Oils: Carrier Oils

Carrier oils, also known as base oils or vegetable oils, are typically thicker than essential oils and facilitate safe delivery of essential oil properties to the scalp and hair. Commonly used carrier oils include coconut, castor, olive, almond, avocado, sunflower, jojoba, and grapeseed oils [3]. Due to the high price of essential oils and potential for skin sensitization, many patients primarily use carrier oils in their hair care regimen. Some of the beneficial nutrients in carrier oils include fatty acids, minerals, and fat-soluble vitamins [12]. Typically applied to the scalp, castor oil can be used to soothe irritation, promote circulation in the scalp and encourages moisture retention in the hair shafts, and is believed to promote hair growth [12]. Jojoba oil decreases scalp dryness and is believed to reduce the appearance of gray hair and promote healthy hair growth [12]. With the exception of coconut oil, there has been limited published research on the beneficial effects of carrier oils on the hair.

Coconut Oil

One of the most commonly used oils for black hair care is coconut oil (Fig. 6.1). Many cultures believe that regular use of coconut oil promotes long healthy hair due to its ability to moisturize the hair instead of just coating it, like other carrier oils [6]. Coconut oil is a triglyceride of lauric acid with a high affinity for hair proteins and is unique, in that it has a low molecular weight and its structure is a straight linear chain [6]. This allows for better absorption and penetration into the hair shaft [6]. Studies investigating the penetrability of sunflower oil have shown that its bulky structure limits its ability to penetrate into the hair fibers, specifically the cortex [6]. Compared to other carrier oils and mineral oil, coconut oil is the only oil that has been shown to decrease protein loss from both damaged and undamaged hair [14]. Coconut oil has been shown to be particularly useful as a prewash treatment. During the washing process, water absorption causes the hair cuticle to repeatedly swell and contract, resulting in damage [6]. By penetrating the hair, coconut oil effectively decreases the amount of swelling and contraction [6]. Although coconut oil's linear chain structure may promote increased absorption, it also responsible for this oils tendency to solidify below 76° Fahrenheit.

Fig. 6.1 Coconut oil is a semisolid at temperatures below 76 °C

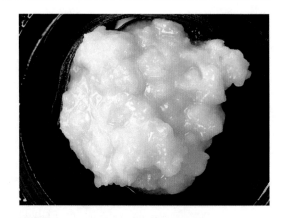

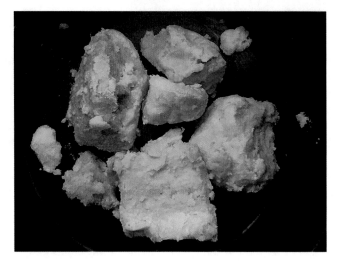

Fig. 6.2 Shea butter

Hair Butters

Hair butters are thick, semisolid products that function as sealants which protect the hair against moisture loss [3]. Shea butter, one of the most widely used butters in black hair care, contains vitamins A, E and essential fatty acids (Fig. 6.2) [12]. Other commonly used butters include mango, cocoa, tucuma, and murumuru. Due to their heavy consistency, they do not spread as easily as oils along hair shafts, therefore they are often whipped or mixed with other ingredients, such as coconut oil, prior to application to the hair.

Aloe Vera Gel and Juice

Aloe vera gel and aloe vera juice are typically extracted from the inside of an aloe vera plant and often used as organic hair conditioners. Aloe vera is primarily composed of water and contains seven of the eight essential amino acids, vitamins A and C, in addition to minerals such as magnesium, zinc, copper, and selenium (Fig. 6.3a, b) [12]. It is believed to hydrate, strengthen, and balance the pH of the hair [3]. Aloe vera gel or juice can be used as a preshampoo treatment, moisturizing shampoo, or conditioner.

Styling Aids

Styling aids are an important component of everyday grooming of black hair. Many of these products are used to create and maintain hairstyles, in addition to moisturizing and protecting the hair. Ingredients commonly found in these products are outlined in Table 6.2.

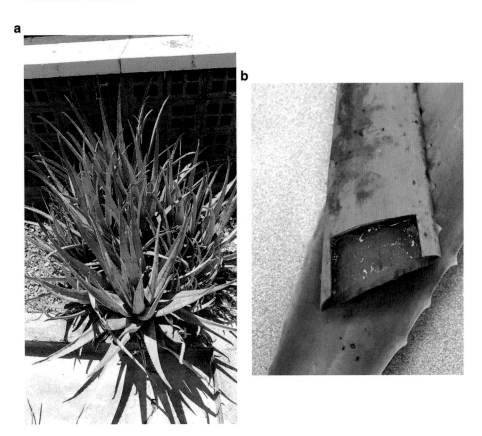

Fig. 6.3 (**a**) Aloe Vera plant, (**b**) Aloe vera leaf cut open to expose aloe vera gel

Table 6.2 Hair care product ingredients and properties

Ingredient	Potential hair benefits	Common identifiers
Humectants	Attract and retain environmental moisture	Glycerin, sodium PCA, panthenol, propylene glycol, sorbitol, sodium lactate
Emollients	Soften and lubricate; help retain moisture	Fats, lanolin, waxes, ceramides, cetyl alcohol
Silicones	Protect against heat damage, detangle, seal in moisture, add shine	Dimethicone, lauryl methicone copolyol, cyclomethicone (contain prefixes PEG- or PPG- and/or suffixes –cone, -conol, -col, and –xane)
Copolymers	Add stiffness to individual hair fibers to maintain hairstyles and control movement	Polyvinylpyrrolidone and vinyl acetate (PVP/MA), Dimethylaminoethylmethacrylate (PVP/DMAEMA)
Cationic polymers/surfactants	Smooth cuticle, soften hair	Polyquaternium
Proteins	Smooth cuticle, strengthen hair, reduce breakage	Collagen, keratin, elastin, hydrolyzed animal and plant proteins
Alcohols	Used as solvents	SD alcohol, isopropyl alcohol

Moisturizing Creams and Lotions

Daily hair moisturizers are typically formulated as lotions (sometimes referred to as "hair milks") or creams that can be applied to the hair regularly. These products are often used to soften the hair, reduce frizz, and add shine. Water-based moisturizers contain water as the first ingredient as well as humectants and fatty alcohols such as cetyl alcohol and ceramides [3]. Oil-based moisturizers usually contain mixtures of petrolatum, lanolin, and mineral oil and are commonly used as "sealants," which trap moisture into the hair shaft and reduce frizz by resisting absorption of external moisture [15].

Gels and Hairsprays

Gels and hairsprays are commonly used to hold the hair in place and increase the longevity of hairstyles. Copolymers are a main ingredient in these products, which can be formulated as aerosolized spray polymers (hairsprays) or clear gel polymers (hair gel) [5]. These products form a protective coating that dries on the hair and can be used to maintain sculpted hairstyles for 1–2 weeks [4].

In addition to maintaining hairstyles, gels are commonly used to flatten or smooth the appearance of tightly curled hair along the hairline in women who chemically or thermally straighten their hair. These products are typically marketed as "edge control" or edge smoothing gels. In women who chemically or thermally straighten their hair, the naturally curly texture of new hair growth is most apparent at the hairline. A process commonly referred to as "smoothing the edges," helps to mask the new growth by allowing the texture at the hairline to match that of the rest of the head. This process involves applying these products to the shorter hairs along the hairline and then brushing this hair in a backward or downward direction to temporarily straighten it.

Although gels and hairsprays may decrease the amount of daily manipulation of the hair, many of these products contain alcohols, which may dry out the hair shaft, making it more fragile and susceptible to breakage [4, 16]. It has been suggested that dermatologists encourage patients to regularly wash these products out of the hair to minimize this drying effect [4].

Setting Lotions/Wrap Foams and Hair Mousse

These liquid or foam-based products are also used to mold and style the hair; however, they offer a lighter, more natural hold than gels and hairsprays [5]. They are typically applied to clean, wet hair, which is then set with rollers or wrapped around the head in a circular fashion. The hair can then be left to air-dry or dried under a hooded dryer.

Silicone-Based Hair Serums

Serums are commonly used as finishing products that add shine and manageability or as prestyling aids that provide heat protection [3]. The primary ingredient in these products is silicone, which is also added to most conditioners and moisturizers to coat the hair and increase moisture retention [17]. By coating and lubricating the hair, silicones decrease friction and allow the hair strands to move easily past one another, thereby protecting against mechanical damage [3]. These products are most commonly used on wet hair to reduce the damage caused by wet combing and detangling. Silicones are also frequently added to thermal protectants, as they decrease the rate of heat transfer from thermal styling appliances to the hair [3].

One of the main disadvantages of silicones is that frequent use can lead to the accumulation of residue on the hair shaft [18]. This buildup weighs the hair down and can prevent moisture absorption by sealing the hair shaft, resulting in dryness and breakage [3]. The amount of buildup is primarily determined by whether the silicone is water soluble or water insoluble [3]. Water-soluble silicones such as dimethicone copolyol and lauryl methicone copolyol provide moisturizing properties and easily break apart in water, leaving behind little residue [3, 17]. These silicones typically contain the prefixes PEG or PPG [3, 17]. Amodimethicone and cyclomethicone are silicones that are not water soluble but have properties that prevent residue accumulation [17]. Water-insoluble silicones create a waterproof coating on the hair shaft and require surfactant-containing shampoos for complete removal [17]. However, these products tend to be effective humidity blockers and shine boosters [3].

Table 6.3 Basic guidelines for choosing hair products

Product type	Most important characteristic	Additional characteristics to consider	Frequency of use
Shampoo	Sulfate free if using regularly	Formulated for color treated or damaged hair if applicable	Every 1–4 times per month depending on hair type. Less often if hair is dry
Rinse-out conditioner	Formulated for dry or damaged hair	Formulated for color treated or damaged hair if applicable	1–3 times per week; more often if hair is dry
Deep Conditioner	Formulated for dry or damaged hair	Formulated for color treated or damaged hair if applicable	1–4 times per month. More often if hair is damaged or dry
Coconut Oil	Should be solid at room temperature, liquid when warmed	None	Before and after every wash; daily as needed for styling
Styler (hair lotion, cream, butter or gel)	None	None	Preferences depend on hair type. Thick butters preferred for thick, dense hair; lotions/milks preferable for fine, thin hair

Selecting Appropriate Hair Products When Transitioning to Natural Hair

For many, the transition to chemical-free natural hair will be their first foray into caring for their own hair on a daily basis. Though this can be an exciting process, it can also be a frustrating process for those who are unfamiliar with the characteristics of their hair. The process of experimenting with different hair products can also be quite expensive, especially in the first months of transitioning. Dermatologists should be sensitive to this issue and when discussing transitioning t o chemical-free styling, this should be acknowledged. The process of selecting products for natural hair can be simplified by focusing on just a handful of cornerstone products for transitioning. Patients should focus only on getting one product of each product type and focus only on the most important characteristics of each product type. These are detailed in Table 6.3.

References

1. Black Consumers and Haircare—US 2015. Available from: http://store.mintel.com/black-consumers-and-haircare-us-august-2015.
2. Roseborough IE, McMichael AJ. Hair care practices in African-American patients. Semin Cutan Med Surg. 2009;28(2):103–8.
3. Davis-Sivasothy A. The science of black hair: a comprehensive guide to textured hair care. Stafford: Saja Publishing; 2011.
4. McMichael AJ. Ethnic hair update: past and present. J Am Acad Dermatol. 2003;48(6 Suppl):S127–33.

5. Draelos ZD. Hair care: an illustrated dermatologic handbook. London: Taylor & Francis; 2005.
6. Rele AS, Mohile RB. Effect of mineral oil, sunflower oil, and coconut oil on prevention of hair damage. J Cosmet Sci. 2003;54(2):175–92.
7. Fregonesi A, Scanavez C, Santos L, De Oliveira A, Roesler R, Escudeiro C, et al. Brazilian oils and butters: the effect of different fatty acid chain composition on human hair physiochemical properties. J Cosmet Sci. 2009;60(2):273–80.
8. Ali B, Al-Wabel NA, Shams S, Ahamad A, Khan SA, Anwar F. Essential oils used in aromatherapy: a systematic review. Asian Pacific J Trop Biomed. 2015;5(8):601–11.
9. al-Sereiti MR, Abu-Amer KM, Sen P. Pharmacology of rosemary (Rosmarinus officinalis Linn.) and its therapeutic potentials. Indian J Exp Biol. 1999;37(2):124–30.
10. Yoon JI, Al-Reza SM, Kang SC. Hair growth promoting effect of Zizyphus jujuba essential oil. Food Chem Toxicol. 2010;48(5):1350–4.
11. Al-Reza SM, Yoon JI, Kim HJ, Kim JS, Kang SC. Anti-inflammatory activity of seed essential oil from Zizyphus jujuba. Food Chem Toxicol. 2010;48(2):639–43.
12. Johnson SA. Evidence-based essential oil therapy: the ultimate guide to the therapeutic and clinical application of essential oils. Orem: Scott A. Johnson Professional Writing Services; 2015.
13. Hay IC, Jamieson M, Ormerod AD. Randomized trial of aromatherapy. Successful treatment for alopecia areata. Arch Dermatol. 1998;134(11):1349–52.
14. Gavazzoni Dias MF. Hair cosmetics: an overview. Int J Trichol. 2015;7(1):2–15.
15. Ruetsch SB, Kamath YK. Effects of thermal treatments with a curling iron on hair fiber. J Cosmet Sci. 2004;55(1):13–27.
16. Callender VD, McMichael AJ, Cohen GF. Medical and surgical therapies for alopecias in black women. Dermatol Ther. 2004;17(2):164–76.
17. Bosley RE, Daveluy S. A primer to natural hair care practices in black patients. Cutis. 2015;95(2):78–80, 106.
18. Crawford K, Hernandez C. A review of hair care products for black individuals. Cutis. 2014;93(6):289–93.

Part III

Ethnic Hair Care: Approach to Developing a Healthy Hair Care Regimen

Developing a Healthy Hair Regimen I: Formulating an Optimal Cleansing and Conditioning Regimen

7

Crystal Aguh

Introduction

Cleansing the hair is the cornerstone of any healthy hair regimen. A typical cleansing routine consists of shampooing the hair, followed by the application of a conditioner. Other important elements include the use of protein-containing conditioners and oils which can further enhance the benefits of routine cleansing. This chapter will provide an in-depth discussion of the role each of these product types plays in maintaining and promoting healthy hair.

Shampoos

Shampooing the hair has many purposes but none greater than cleansing the scalp of buildup such as dirt and oil. Modern shampoos contain many ingredients designed to effectively cleanse the hair and scalp while also producing the luster and shine that many consumers crave. Shampoos work to weaken the forces that bind dirt and residue to the hair as well as remove buildup of hair products and sebum [1]. Sebum, the product of the scalp's sebaceous glands, is a natural moisturizing oil that traverses down the hair shaft [2]. This serves to protect the shaft from damage and provide a natural shine [3]. However, accumulation of excess sebum can give the hair an oily appearance, which may be undesirable, particularly in individuals with straight hair who experience rapid movement of sebum from the root to tips [3]. Sebum is also a potent attractant of dirt, dust, and other pollutants from the environment [2].

C. Aguh, M.D. (✉)
Department of Dermatology, Johns Hopkins University School of Medicine,
5200 Eastern Avenue, Suite 2500, Baltimore, MD 21224, USA

© Springer International Publishing Switzerland 2017   79
C. Aguh, G.A. Okoye (eds.), *Fundamentals of Ethnic Hair*,
DOI 10.1007/978-3-319-45695-9_7

Though there is likely no difference in the sebum production between racial groups, it is more difficult for sebum to coat the entire length of very curly hair. This is one of the reasons that curly hair types are more prone to damage from routine grooming [1, 4]. For this reason, frequent removal of sebum is undesirable, and frequent shampooing can result in hair that appears excessively dry, dull, and lifeless [5].

Recommendations for Shampooing Frequency

Many patients will inquire about the ideal frequency of washing, but this varies based on the individual. For patients with a history of seborrheic dermatitis, more frequent washing alone may lead to improvement of symptoms [6]. In general, shampooing may lead to decreased inflammation on the scalp, but may be more damaging to the hair shaft due to its ability to strip the hair of sebum [3, 7]. For this reason, those with dry or curly hair may benefit from avoiding frequent shampooing. The frequency of hair washing in those with curly hair can vary widely from once weekly to once monthly depending on the initial condition of the hair. To minimize risk of damage, shampoo should be focused mostly on the scalp to help remove sebum and the user should allow water to gently rinse the shampoo down the hair shaft [3] (Fig. 7.1). Additional considerations related to shampoo ingredients are discussed later.

Fig. 7.1 Shampooing the hair

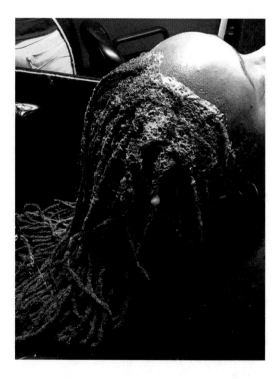

Shampoo Ingredients

Shampoos are formulated with special detergents aimed at uniquely expelling dirt and oils from the hair shaft without damaging the shaft or leaving behind calcified buildup [1–3]. Shampoos work by decreasing the surface tensions between water and dirt allowing the dirt to be washed away during the cleansing process [6]. The first shampoos were formulated like traditional soaps and resulted in the buildup of calcified salts, particularly when used in hard water [2]. Modern shampoos are formulated with surface active ingredients, or surfactants, that are able to work well in all types of water [2]. Surfactants consist of a lipophilic group, which attracts oil and dirt, and a hydrophilic group, which attracts water. They are classified according to the charge of their hydrophilic group [2, 3, 6].

Anionic Surfactants

The most common type of surfactant used in shampoos is anionic surfactants [1, 3]. Anionic surfactants contain a negatively charged hydrophilic group and are considered to be the most effective at removing sebum when compared to other classes of surfactants [3, 8]. Examples of anionic surfactants include lauryl sulfates, laureth sulfates, sarcosinates, and sulfosuccinates [8]. These ingredients are particularly effective at creating a rich lather which can be important to consumers who, though falsely, may equate effective cleansing with lathering ability [5]. Sodium lauryl sulfate (SLS) is the most effective at removing sebum but is harsh to the hair, thus this ingredient is typically used in shampoos marketed to those with oily hair [3]. Sodium laureth sulfates (SLES) are less harsh to the hair than SLS but are also quite effective at removing sebum [9]. The use of shampoos containing anionic surfactants can be beneficial when there is excess product buildup but should be limited to 1–2 times per month for those with curly hair. However, for more routine use, shampoos containing anionic surfactants should be avoided in those with dry or curly hair.

When consumers refer to "sulfate-free" shampoos, they are generally referring to shampoos that are free of anionic surfactants [1]. Though anionic surfactants are effective at cleansing the hair, they can often leave the hair dry and more prone to breakage. For those with very curly hair, overcleansing can be particularly damaging due to the decreased sebum content along the length of the hair strand. As a result, sulfate-free shampoos have become increasingly popular for use in curly hair, as well as other hair types that are prone to dryness. Patients should be cautioned, however, that this term is defined quite loosely and shampoos may still contain drying anionic surfactants even if they do not contain traditional sulfate-based surfactants like SLS (Table 7.1).

Cationic Surfactants

Cationic surfactants are differentiated by their positively charged hydrophilic group [1, 2, 6, 9]. Unlike anionic surfactants, cationic surfactants increase the softness and manageability of the hair [2, 3, 6]. Cationic surfactants are particularly attracted to negatively charged acids, which are abundant in damaged hair. As a result, these surfactants are particularly effective for those with dry, damaged hair [6].

Table 7.1 Shampoo recommendations for curly, dry, or damaged hair

Non anionic "sulfate-free" surfactants	Anionic surfactants
Less drying than anionic surfactants; ideal for regular use especially in curly/kinky hair	*The products remove product buildup but can be drying. Use sparingly*
Benzalkonium Chloride	Sodium Lauryl Sulfate
Cetrimonium Chloride	Sodium Laureth Sulfate
Cocamidopropyl Betaine	Sodium Lauroyl Sarcosinate
Decyl Glucoside	Ammonium Lauryl Sulfate
Lauryl Glucoside	Sodium Myreth Sulfate
Stearamidopropyl Dimethylamine	Sodium C14-16 Olefin Sulfonate
Cocamide MEA	Disodium laureth sulfosuccinate
Disodium Cocoamphodipropionate	
Behentrimonium Methosulfate	

Common cationic surfactants include quaternary ammonium salts such as benzalkonium chloride and cetrimonium chloride [5]. Behentrimonium methosulfate is another example of a cationic surfactant, and despite having 'sulfate' within its name, is a moisturizing ingredient found in sulfate-free shampoo formulations. Despite their ability to add softness to the hair, the use of cationic surfactants in shampoos is limited because they cannot be combined with negatively charged anionic surfactants as this combination results in shampoos with minimal cleansing ability [3].

Amphoteric Surfactants

Amphoteric surfactants contain both an anionic group and a cationic group resulting in a neutrally charged surfactant with moderate cleansing ability [8]. Amphoteric surfactants operate as a cationic surfactant in low, acidic pH environments and as an anionic surfactant in more basic, high pH environments [2, 3, 6]. These surfactants also improve manageability and are found in many sulfate-free shampoo formulations. They can be combined with anionic surfactants to help increase cleansing ability. Amphoteric surfactants are also the most common type of detergent used in baby shampoos due to their gentle nature and ability to partially anesthetize the eye to minimize irritation [3]. Common amphoteric surfactants include betaines, sultaines, and imidazoliums [2].

Nonionic Surfactants

Unlike the previously mentioned surfactants, nonionic surfactants contain no polar groups and are compatible with all other surfactant types [2, 3, 6]. They are the mildest of all of the surfactants and leave the hair manageable [3]. They are often combined with cationic or anionic surfactants but can be used alone in shampoo formulations that are designed to be gentle to the hair [2, 6]. These ingredients are especially popular in shampoos formulated for natural black hair but can be used in all hair types, particularly in those individuals who have damaged, dry, or color-treated hair. Examples of nonionic surfactants include decyl glucoside, fatty alcohol ethoxylates (such as cetyl alcohol and stearyl alcohol), and sorbitan ether esters [2, 3, 6]

Shampoo Additives

Shampoos contain several additives that are designed to improve its appeal to consumers, many of which are not related to its cleansing ability. Conditioning agents, which are discussed in detail later, are often added to shampoos to impart softness to the hair as harsh surfactants can cause the hair to appear dry and lifeless [8]. Thickening agents are also often added to shampoos since thicker shampoos are perceived as being more effective at cleansing. Similarly, opacifiers are added to create the illusion of a pearly sheen, which also increases the esthetic appeal of a shampoo. Lastly, sequestering agents are added to shampoos to prevent buildup of calcium and magnesium ions on the hair which cause the hair to appear dull [2, 8].

Shampoo pH is another important factor to consider, as alkaline shampoos with a pH greater than 7 can increase frizz and worsen manageability [10]. This occurs because alkaline shampoos increase the negative charge on the hair, the same negative charge that conditioners aim to combat. Alkaline shampoos can also increase hair swelling and subsequent damage. When shampoo pH is decreased to acidic levels, manageability is improved; some shampoos add ingredients such as glycolic acid or other acidic ingredients to lower the pH [9]. Interestingly, most commercial shampoos are alkaline in nature but salon-grade shampoos are more likely to maintain a pH <5.0 [10].

Preshampoo Treatments

Applying oil to the hair prior to shampooing has been shown to decrease swelling of the cuticle, which can in turn prevent damage during grooming of wet hair [11]. Repeated swelling and drying, termed hygral fatigue, is a common cause of hair damage [1]. Coconut oil has been the most well-studied oil shown to prevent damage to the hair that occurs as a result of hygral fatigue [11, 12]. Coconut oil, which is polar and hydrophobic, has a high affinity for the cortex of the hair shaft, allowing it to penetrate more deeply and prevent hair swelling by blocking water entry. In one study, coconut oil was shown to reduce cuticular swelling by 48% compared to untreated hair [11]. Mineral oil also has the ability to decrease swelling due to its hydrophobicity but cannot penetrate the shaft as deeply due to its higher molecular weight and its lack of polarity [11]. Applying oils to the hair prior to shampooing is commonly termed 'prepooing', which is a shortened form of 'preshampooing'. Regular prewash application of oils to the hair is recommended for those with dry or damaged hair (Table 7.2).

Conditioners

Because hair is nonliving, total repair of the hair shaft is not possible and one can only hope to minimize further damage through a healthy hair regimen [13]. Repeated use of heat, bleach, routine grooming, and/or chemical processing can lead to weathered hair which manifests as tangling, frizzing, and hair breakage [1].

Table 7.2 Shampooing tips for dry/damaged or naturally curly hair

Eliminate or minimize use of shampoos containing anionic surfactants
Shampoo only when necessary for removal of product or sebum buildup
Direct shampoo to scalp only and allow water to rinse shampoo along shaft
Apply a moisturizing oil such as coconut oil to the hair shaft prior to shampooing

Conditioners have the ability to temporarily repair dry damaged hair as well as prevent future damage and this makes it even more important to routine hair care than shampooing [13, 14]. Routine grooming of black hair is more likely to result in frayed, split ends than in other racial groups making prevention of damage through use of conditioners especially important [15]. However, the essentials of a hair care regimen for dry, damaged Caucasian or Asian hair is quite similar to black hair and reliance on conditioners should be the cornerstone of a healthy hair regimen regardless of racial background.

Sebum is the ideal hair conditioner but has difficulty traveling the length of the hair shaft in curly or kinky hair [3]. Conditioners are formulated to mimic the action of sebum on the hair but have the added benefit of being applied directly to the length of the hair shaft by the user. Conditioners can also improve frizz and minimize flyaways. Flyaways are a result of static electricity between hair strands and are particularly noticeable in dry hair. By increasing hair moisture, the friction between hair strands is decreased, and hair is more manageable [5, 13].

Split ends, also known as trichoptilosis, occur as a result of frequent trauma to the hair shaft. This leads to the absence of the protective cuticle, leaving the cortex and medulla exposed. Conditioners also have the ability to temporarily mend split ends by realigning the cortex and medulla to halt further damage [3]. Conditioners come in many different formulations depending on the desired effect and are described in detail later.

Rinse-out Conditioners

These conditioners are meant to be applied to the hair immediately after shampooing to help balance out any dryness created as a result of shampoo use. The most common conditioning agents are quaternary ammonium compounds, which are positively charged cationic compounds that balance out the anionic charge of shampoos [1]. In addition to increasing manageability as noted earlier, these conditioners also flatten the scales of the hair cuticle, increasing the shine and luster of the hair [3]. However, because they are rinsed out immediately, they are less effective at repairing hair damage than other conditioner types that have prolonged contact with the hair shaft [3].

Examples of quaternary ammonium compounds include behentrimonium chloride and stearalkonium chloride. Many conditioners also contain silicone, a potent moisturizing agent that help imparts softness to the hair. Silicones, however, are water resistant and thus can leave a thin film on the hair after rinsing [3].

Deep Conditioners

While rinse-out conditioners are meant to be rinsed instantly, deep conditioners are typically left on the hair for at least ten minutes to allow for prolonged contact with the hair shaft. Deep conditioners, also called hair 'masks/masques' are typically thick creams that are most effective when used on very damaged, weathered hair [2]. For those with extensive damage as a result of chemical processing or grooming, deep conditioners can temporarily reverse the drying effects associated with permanent damage and can be used weekly [2]. These conditioners typically contain higher amounts of quaternary conditioners in addition to protein-containing conditioners which serve to moisturize and strengthen the hair, respectively [3]. Deep conditioners are often applied with heat as heat lifts the cuticular scales allowing for deeper penetration of the conditioner [3]. Additionally, deep conditioners can be mixed with oils to improve the overall feel and appearance of the hair.

Leave-in Conditioners

These conditioners are particularly popular among those with curly, kinky hair. Leave-in conditioners are designed to be applied following the use of shampoos and conditioners but are not meant to be rinsed out. They typically contain conditioning agents such as silicones, humectants, such as glycerin, or film-forming agents. Film-forming agents are lightweight polymers that are designed to coat the hair and fill in hair shaft defects, and can also function to eliminate static electricity [3]. Leave-in conditioners can be applied daily to aid in styling and prevent damage from routine grooming.

Protein-Containing Conditioners

Protein-containing conditioners can be formulated as rinse-out, deep, or leave-in conditioners; however, they are most effective when maintaining prolonged contact with the hair as seen in the latter two formulations [3]. These are considered essential to the regimen of patients with dry and/or damaged hair. Over time, damaging habits such as coloring, heat application, chemical processing, and routine grooming can lead to flattening of the cuticular scales and the creation of holes within the shaft (see Chap. 3). This leads to decreased strength in the hair shaft and makes the hair more prone to damage. Hydrolyzed proteins are small enough to enter the hair shaft and repair these holes to increase the strength of the hair shaft by up to 10 % [3]. This benefit, however, only lasts until the following shampooing as the excess protein is washed away.

Conditioner-Only Washing

Conditioner-only washing (called "cowashing") is an option for those who prefer to avoid shampooing altogether. This method of washing has recently become more popular particularly in those with naturally curly or kinky hair. Shampooing is more damaging to the hair shaft than beneficial and is truly only required when residue buildup is significant [8]. In patients with low sebum content along the hair shaft, frequent shampooing is likely unnecessary and less important than conditioning which has the ability to repair the hair, as previously discussed. Rinse-out conditioners are most commonly used for conditioner-only washing in contrast to deep conditioners, which are more likely to leave an undesirable film on the hair. However, with repeated use rinse-out conditioners will also leave an accumulation of film on the hair, necessitating the use of a traditional shampoo at least once or twice monthly to prevent limp, dull hair from product buildup. Conditioners marketed as 'cowash' conditioners commonly contain nonionic surfactants, amphoteric surfactants, and/or quaternary conditioning agents. Because washing with conditioners alone is less damaging to the shaft than shampooing, some with curly hair may elect to cowash daily or several times a week particularly those who live in dry climates.

Protein Treatments

The cortex of the hair is responsible for tensile strength and makes up a majority of the hair shaft [16]. The cells of the cortex are comprised of a sulfur protein matrix and keratin filaments which are lost when the hair becomes damaged [16]. While thin, fine strands are more susceptible to damage, all hair types are at risk for substantial damage as a result of traumatizing hair practices. Hydrolyzed proteins have been shown to protect the hair from damage and when added to cleansers and can also improve the shine, gloss, and softness of the hair [17]. These proteins are hydrolyzed to a small molecular weight to allow for penetration of the hair shaft [3]. In doing so, these proteins can patch defects within the hair shaft and increase the overall strength [3].

Similar to protein conditioners, protein treatments are specialized products marketed toward those with severely damaged hair and often contain conditioning agents as well. Most treatments are designed to remain on the hair for at least ten minutes to maximize benefit. Studies have shown that the greatest amount of protein is absorbed within the first fifteen minutes of application when applied with water [17]. Protein absorption is particularly increased in hair that is more severely damaged, which has more defects to fill than normal, undamaged hair [17]. These treatments are typically used on a monthly or bimonthly basis as many consumers will report dryness and brittleness with overusage of these protein-containing products. Examples of hydrolyzed proteins commonly used in hair products include keratin, collagen, and elastin [3, 17].

Soak and Smear Repurposed

The "soak and smear" is a popular technique used by dermatologists to treat severe eczema, a skin condition characterized by pruritus, dry skin, and a defective skin barrier [18]. Patients are instructed to soak their skin in water for at least 20 min and follow with the application a thick emollient, usually petrolatum or a medicated steroid ointment [18]. In the skin, this technique works quite well to help trap moisture while also allowing for deeper penetration of the medication.

A similar process can be used for the hair to aid in moisture retention. As previously noted, dry hair is more prone to breakage and is more difficult to style [3, 15]. Increased hair moisture results in fewer tangles and increased hair elasticity enhancing combability and styling ease [3]. When applied to wet hair, some oils such as coconut oil have been shown to decrease moisture loss and aid in moisture retention [19]. Coconut oil has also been shown to decrease protein loss when used as a postwash treatment thus magnifying its benefit when used in this method [12].

The repurposed soak and smear method for the hair is as follows:

1. Shampoo and condition hair per routine
2. Lightly blot the hair with a towel
3. Apply a water-based leave-in conditioner to the hair
4. Follow immediately with a hair oil (such as coconut oil, olive oil, jojoba oil, etc.)
5. Air dry and style as desired

This method is popularly referred to as the "L.O.C." method in natural black hair care forums and websites which stands for 'liquid, oil, cream' as some have noticed added benefit by following oil application with thick butters or creams that do not contain water as primary ingredients. Instead, these butters contain more conditioning agents and act similar to emollients. Occlusive moisturizers such as petrolatum and mineral oil are particularly effective at preventing water loss in the skin and are often found in ethnic hair care products as well [20]. Products containing these ingredients can also be used after oils but may leave the hair feeling excessively greasy or limp.

This repurposed soak and smear method can be executed as often as needed throughout the week. In fact, for those not wishing to shampoo/condition prior to applying oils, water can be sprayed directly onto the hair shaft until damp to create a similar result.

Conclusion

The cleansing routine is critically important to maintaining the health of the hair. Hair that has been chemically processed is chronically dry or is experiencing recurrent breakage will benefit most from the use of gentle, sulfate-free cleansers and the

Table 7.3 Cleansing and conditioning recommendations

Shampoo is effective at cleansing the scalp of buildup but can strip the hair shaft of protective sebum. Patients with dry or damaged hair may benefit from less frequent shampooing or shampoos containing mild surfactants

Conditioners should be a cornerstone of any hair care regimen for naturally curly or damaged hair as they have the ability to prevent future damage

Applying oils prior to shampooing can protect the hair from hygral fatigue and damage that occurs from routine washing

Protein has the ability to temporarily repair damaged hair shafts. Regular protein treatments are advisable in those with severe damage from grooming or chemical processing

The "Soak and Smear" method can be applied to hair to aid in moisture retention for those with dry hair

use of protein-containing conditioners. For a more detailed list of cleansing recommendations, please see Table 7.3.

References

1. Gavazzoni Dias MF. Hair cosmetics: an overview. Int J Trichol. 2015;7(1):2–15.
2. Bouillon C. Shampoos and hair conditioners. Clin Dermatol. 1988;6(3):83–92.
3. Draelos ZD. Hair care: an illustrated dermatologic handbook. London: CRC Press; 2004.
4. Taylor SC. Skin of color: biology, structure, function, and implications for dermatologic disease. J Am Acad Dermatol. 2002;46(2):S41–62.
5. Draelos ZD. The biology of hair care. Dermatol Clin. 2000;18(4):651–8.
6. Trueb RM. Shampoos: ingredients, efficacy and adverse effects. J Dtsch Dermatol Ges. 2007;5(5):356–65.
7. Beach RA, Wilkinson KA, Gumedze F, Khumalo NP. Baseline sebum IL-1alpha is higher than expected in afro-textured hair: a risk factor for hair loss? J Cosmet Dermatol. 2012;11(1):9–16.
8. Draelos ZD. Essentials of hair care often neglected: hair cleansing. Int J Trichol. 2010;2(1):24–9.
9. Draelos ZD. Shampoos, conditioners, and camouflage techniques. Dermatol Clin. 2013;31(1):173–8.
10. Gavazzoni Dias MF, de Almeida AM, Cecato PM, Adriano AR, Pichler J. The shampoo pH can affect the hair: myth or reality? Int J Trichol. 2014;6(3):95–9.
11. Ruetsch SB, Kamath YK, Rele AS, Mohile RB. Secondary ion mass spectrometric investigation of penetration of coconut and mineral oils into human hair fibers: relevance to hair damage. J Cosmet Sci. 2001;52(3):169–84.
12. Rele AS, Mohile RB. Effect of mineral oil, sunflower oil, and coconut oil on prevention of hair damage. J Cosmet Sci. 2003;54(2):175–92.
13. Bhushan B, Wei G, Haddad P. Friction and wear studies of human hair and skin. Wear. 2005;259(7):1012–21.
14. Ruetsch SB, Kamath YK, Kintrup L, Schwark HJ. Effects of conditioners on surface hardness of hair fibers: an investigation using atomic force microscopy. J Cosmet Sci. 2003;54(6):579–88.
15. Khumalo NP, Doe PT, Dawber RP, Ferguson DJ. What is normal black African hair? A light and scanning electron-microscopic study. J Am Acad Dermatol. 2000;43(5 Pt 1):814–20.
16. Bolduc C, Shapiro J. Hair care products: waving, straightening, conditioning, and coloring. Clin Dermatol. 2001;19(4):431–6.
17. Ścibisz M, Arct J, Pytkowska K. Protein hydrolysates in cosmetics production, part II. SÖFW J Wydanie Polskie. 2008;4:12–9.

18. Gutman AB, Kligman AM, Sciacca J, James WD. Soak and smear: a standard technique revisited. Arch Dermatol. 2005;141(12):1556–9.
19. Keis K, Huemmer CL, Kamath YK. Effect of oil films on moisture vapor absorption on human hair. J Cosmet Sci. 2007;58(2):135–45.
20. Draelos ZD. Therapeutic moisturizers. Dermatol Clin. 2000;18(4):597–607.

Developing a Healthy Hair Regimen II: Transitioning to Chemical-Free Styling (To Natural Hair) and Prevention of Hair Trauma

8

Rawn E. Bosley, Chelsea Rain St. Claire, and Kayla St. Claire

Introduction

The term "natural" is used to describe chemical-free hair styling in people of African descent and others with naturally curly hair (Fig. 8.1a, b). The natural hair renaissance in people of African, African-American, Afro-Caribbean, and Afro-Latina descent has swept across American culture. Images of women of color with their natural hair have infiltrated popular culture in various aspects of television, film, advertising, and social media. As the natural hair phenomenon continues to be woven into popular culture, product development targeting natural hair styling has expanded vastly. Sales of chemical products such as relaxers have declined while the sale of styling products such as moisturizers and curl creams has soared. The hair care industry has increased marketing of natural hair products to satisfy the growing demand. Major brands have not only created product lines dedicated to black hair but have also reformulated established products with ingredients that natural hair enthusiasts look for in their hair care products. Sales of styling products are projected to reach $1.4 billion by 2020 [1] (Fig. 8.2). As the United States becomes increasingly diverse, dermatologists will benefit from knowing how to address the needs of patients seeking assistance with transitioning to and maintaining natural hairstyles.

R.E. Bosley, M.D. (✉)
Doctor's Approach Dermatology & Surgery, 2685 Jolly Rd., Okemos, MI 48864, USA

C.R.S. Claire, B.S.
Michigan State College of Human Medicine,
15 Michigan St. NE, Grand Rapids, MI 49503, USA

K.S. Claire, B.A.
University of Illinois at Chicago College of Medicine,
808 S Wood St., Chicago, IL 60612, USA

© Springer International Publishing Switzerland 2017
C. Aguh, G.A. Okoye (eds.), *Fundamentals of Ethnic Hair*,
DOI 10.1007/978-3-319-45695-9_8

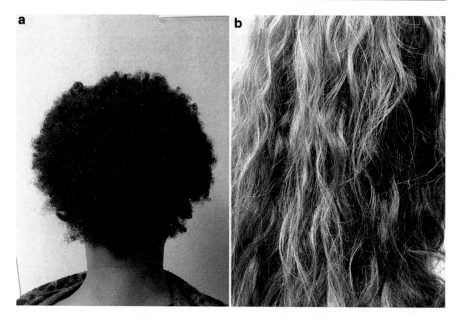

Fig. 8.1 (**a**) Image of tightly curled hair most commonly seen in people of African descent vs. (**b**) loose waves seen more commonly in Caucasians

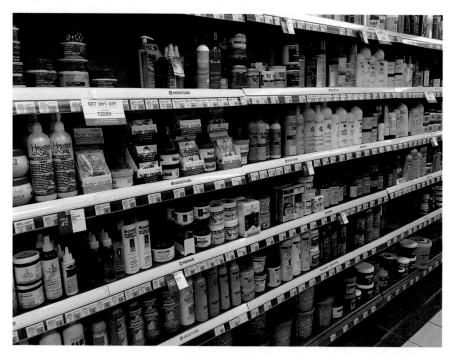

Fig. 8.2 A beauty supply aisle dedicated to natural hair products

Since the early twentieth century, chemical relaxers and thermal straightening methods have been popular hair care techniques in people of African descent. These popular hair care practices, when used excessively or inappropriately may lead to hair damage. Though the etiologies of common scalp and hair disorders in various ethnic groups are multifactorial, traumatic hair styling practices are often implicated as cause of hair loss, which is the 4th most common dermatologic condition in African-American patients [2, 3]. As patients seek medical care for these conditions, dermatologists and other hair care professionals often recommend the cessation of traumatic hair styling for less traumatic and damaging natural hairstyles. Additionally, patients should seek consultation with hair care professionals that are familiar with natural hairstyling.

Unique Properties of Curly Hair

It is important for dermatologists and hair care professionals to understand the unique properties of curly hair, as discussed in Chap. 1. Curly hair is more susceptible to damage due to increased mechanical fragility, and the propensity of the hair to form knots (trichonodosis) and split ends (trichoptilosis) [4]. Forceful manipulation of the hair with brushing or combing may cause additional fracturing of the hair. For this reason, frequent use of combs and brushes should be discouraged. Additionally, straight hair is more easily coated with sebum and therefore are less likely to fracture from excessive dryness [5].

Hair Porosity

Porosity is the hair's ability to absorb and retain moisture. The hair cuticle acts as a protective barrier to the inner components of the hair shaft. The cuticle also determines the hair's ability to allow moisture to be drawn into the interior of the hair shaft. The cuticle can be damaged by overmanipulation of the hair, exposure to heat, or humidity as well as exposure to chemicals.

Determining Hair Porosity

The porosity of the hair can be determined by the use of several simple tests. The most commonly performed test is the water or float test. For this test a few strands of clean hair can be placed in a bowl or large cup of water. The hair should be placed in water for several minutes. For low porosity hair, the hair will float. Conversely, highly porous hair will quickly sink into the water. Hair with normal or medium porosity will float before gradually sinking over several minutes. Another way to measure porosity is to slide the fingers up the hair shaft toward the scalp. In low porosity hair, the hair shaft feels smooth whereas high porosity hair feels rough or bumpy. Lastly, porosity can be measured by spraying a small amount of water onto the hair. In low porosity hair, water is poorly absorbed and beads upon the hair. In contrast, highly porous hair will quickly absorb the water [6].

Recommended Products for Low Porosity Hair

Hair with low porosity resists moisture and may lead to the buildup of thick or protein-rich products. The use of these products in low porosity hair can lead to hair damage due to excessive buildup and the need to repeatedly wash the hair with harsh sulfate-containing shampoos to remove residue. Those with low porosity hair should use products that are lighter and contain humectants to encourage the absorption of moisture. Commonly used humectants in hair products include glycerin, propylene glycol, honey, and sorbitol (see Chap. 6) [7]. Hydrolyzed proteins are less likely to buildup on the hair and can be used in this hair type. Products for low porosity hair commonly contain light oils and emollients such as argan oil, jojoba oil, and coconut oil. The use of low to moderate heat hair steamers and dryers while conditioning can open the hair cuticle to allow moisture uptake [7].

Recommended Products for Normal Porosity Hair

In general, normal or medium porosity hair is more easily maintained compared to the other types. The hair cuticle typically functions properly to retain moisture and prevent the excessive release of moisture. Similar to low porosity products, normal porosity hair products are liquid-based conditioners such as milks and creams as well as oils and butters. Protein-containing conditioners can be used occasionally to maintain medium porosity hair [6]. Though heat can be helpful when conditioning, it is not essential to uptake of the conditioning product.

Recommended Products for High Porosity Hair

High porosity hair can occur as a result of external damage to the hair cuticle from chemicals and heat or it can be an intrinsic property of an individual's hair. Damage to the hair cuticle allows absorption of too much moisture into the hair. Excessive moisture can cause hair swelling resulting in tangling, frizziness, and fracturing of the hair. Additionally, highly porous hair cannot retain moisture, leading to dry and fragile hair. The key to managing highly porous hair is to use products that will maintain or lock in moisture. Combining a leave-in conditioner and a viscous oil or heavy butter such as castor oil, olive oil, or cocoa butter seals the hair cuticle and prevents moisture loss [7]. Products used for high porosity hair should contain lower concentrations of humectants to discourage excessive absorption of moisture, especially in humid environments.

Role of Dermatologic Assessment in Transitioning to Natural Hair

Relaxer use is very common among black women. In one study in the US, 91 % of patients presenting to a dermatologist for evaluation of scarring hair loss regularly used a relaxer [8]. Therefore, dermatologists should be prepared to discuss the pros and cons of relaxer use in these patients and the role of chemical-free styling in the management of their hair loss (see Chapter 2) [8]. Additionally, management of underlying dermatologic disease and understanding the patient's' current hairstyling regimen may be necessary in aiding patients' transition to chemical-free hair styling. For example, dandruff and seborrheic dermatitis (see Chap. 9) are common in black women and, if present, may influence the types of styling products used in patients transitioning to chemical-free styling (see Chap. 6). Additionally, when patients have transitioned to natural hair, their preferences for topical medication vehicles may change. For instance, ointment-based topical medications are generally preferred over water-based products in people with natural hair.

For black women, transitioning to chemical-free hairstyling can be a difficult and emotional experience. These seemingly minor considerations can go a long way to building patient trust and easing an otherwise difficult transition.

Going Natural: "Transitioning" vs. "The Big Chop"

Patients may decide to completely cut off the chemically treated hair, commonly known as "the big chop" (Fig. 8.3). The hair is cut down to the untreated natural hair, also known as "new growth." The "new growth" represents the hair growth since the last chemical relaxer. Patients are then left with much shorter hair. For patients who decide against the "big chop," other methods can be used for a more gradual "transitioning" phase. These include using protective or low

Fig. 8.3 A patient one week after her 'big chop'

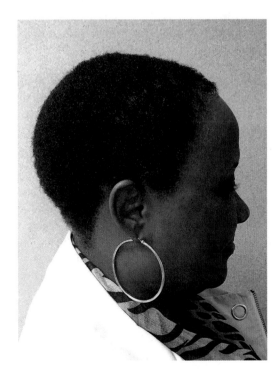

manipulation styling such as braids, wigs, or weaves, and gradually trimming the chemically treated hair as the new growth continues to lengthen. As natural hair growth occurs during the transitioning period, patients will experience varying hair textures, which may cause matting and tangling. The area of the hair where the two different textures meet is known as the "line of demarcation." Patients should be advised that if they decide to use the "transitioning" method they should avoid the temptation of using thermal tools to make their curly hair match their straight, chemically treated hair. Over time, the repeated use of thermal styling tools leads to damage and breakage. Cleansing, conditioning, and daily moisturizing are important aspects of transitioning and styling natural hair. For details and product/ingredient recommendations, see Chap. 6.

Protective Styling

Protective hairstyles are styles that hide the ends of the hair, thus allowing the hair to be protected from damage. Protective styles include hair braiding, twists, weaves, and wigs. These styles allow the hair to be easily styled while new hair growth develops [9]. These styles have the benefit of being worn for weeks to months enabling hair growth while simultaneously avoiding breakage and shedding as a result of daily grooming and manipulation. For a more detailed discussion on the installation of wigs and weaves, please see Chapter 5.

One of the disadvantages of protective styles is that the patient's hair cannot be washed as often. This leads to dry, brittle hair that is prone to breakage. Additionally, wearing extensions for extended periods of time can also lead to breakage (see Chap. 5). Patients should be reminded to moisturize their hair often if they choose to transition to natural hair in this way. Patients must be reminded of the primary purpose of the protective styles. Excessively heavy hair may pull on the patient's hair weakening the single stands or loosening underlying braids causing breakage. Leaving these styles in place for more than 6 to 8 weeks could have deleterious effects on the hair.

Low Manipulation Styling

Low manipulation styles, in contrast to protective hairstyles, do not require the end of the hair to be tucked away. These styles are relatively simple and require less styling and manipulation in the form of brushing, combing, or detangling. The premise behind low manipulation styles is that decreased frequency of daily grooming will prevent unnecessary damage, leading to retained hair length. Examples of low manipulation styles include wash and go (Fig. 8.4a, b), buns (Fig. 8.5), bantu knot outs (Fig. 8.6a, b), or roller sets. Additional benefits of low manipulation styles include easier access to the hair for cleansing and conditioning.

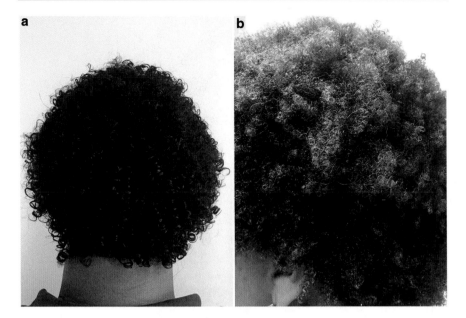

Fig. 8.4   A wash and go on (**a**) curly hair and (**b**) kinky hair

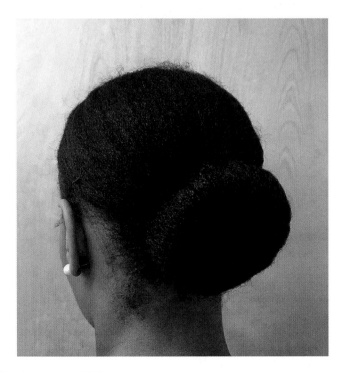

Fig. 8.5   Low bun on natural hair

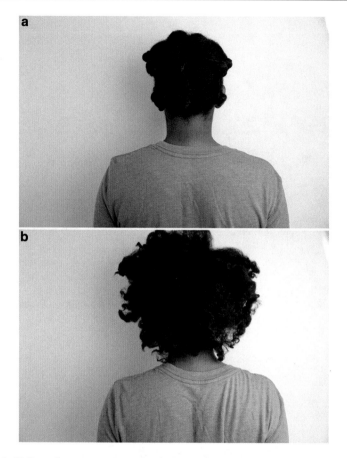

Fig. 8.6 (**a**, **b**) Bantu knot-out, an example of a low manipulation hair style

Daily Grooming Recommendations

Whether patients are using protective styles or low manipulation styles, care must be taken to avoid tangling of the hair. Mismanagement of tangled hair can lead to hair breakage, as hair at the line of demarcation is often very brittle. Manually detangling with the fingers or wide tooth combs from the hair ends to the root is the proper method to detangle hair (Fig. 8.7). The use of detangling conditioners may aid in this process. Regular trimming of the hair can prevent the hair from tangling and halt the progression of split ends traveling up the hair shaft. The hair should be trimmed every 2–4 months depending on the amount of breakage. Another important aspect in preventing matting and tangling of the hair is to decrease the amount of friction on the hair. Braiding or twisting the

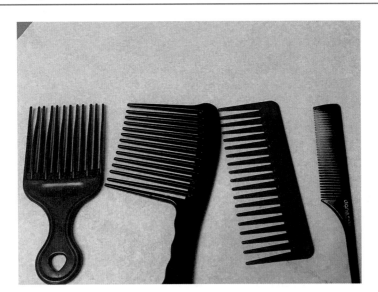

Fig. 8.7 Variety of combs from left to right: afro pick, wide tooth comb, wide tooth comb, rat tail comb

hair into a lengthened state to prevent the hair from curling upon itself and kinking can help decrease friction on the hair. Other methods to decrease the amount of friction on the hair include wearing silk bonnets and/or using satin pillowcases while sleeping. Pulling the hair up into a loose ponytail at the top of the head or "pineappling" the hair at night can decrease the amount of tangling and protect the curl of the hair [9].

Conclusion

In conclusion, transitioning to chemical-free styling can be difficult but there are many benefits, especially for people with hair and scalp disorders. Dermatologists can play a critical role in this process by educating themselves about natural hair management and by working alongside hair stylists to develop an optimal hair styling regimen (Table 8.1). Many patients look to online resources to provide insight into how to maintain healthy hair (Table 8.2). In addition to staying abreast of new evidence-based medical research on the evaluation and treatment of hair and scalp diseases, dermatologists should also be aware of these online resources for patients who need more information about natural hair care.

Table 8.1 Summary of recommendations for natural hair styling

Dermatologists should discuss the benefits of natural hair styling in patients with hair and scalp disease

Avoid frequent use of combs and brushes to minimize risk of trauma to the hair

Use of protective styles such as weaves, wigs, and extensions can aid in transitioning to natural hair and protect the hair from breakage

Low manipulation styles avoid the use of frequent brushing or combing thus minimizing trauma and maximizing hair growth

Dermatologists should consider the vehicle of prescription medication in patients with natural hair

Table 8.2 Patient perspective—healthy hair practices

Growing up I wanted long hair like every other girl I knew at the time, but I always assumed it was determined by elements beyond my control. Some girls have long hair, some don't and that was that. Of course I still longed for hair flowing down my back, but truth be told I felt lucky to at least have hair down to my shoulders. Once I was old enough to get a relaxer, I was at the hair salon every other week getting my hair done. I had the same lovely woman do my hair all the way through high school and even when I was away at college I quickly found a trusted stylist to do my hair when I needed it relaxed. After college I moved around quite a bit and found myself testing out several different hair salons. Without realizing it somewhere in there my hair got shorter and thinner than it once was.

At this point I was fed up with hair salons in general. The last stylist that I went to told me that my hair was badly damaged, she gave me a trim and told me that I would need a protein treatment with my next appointment. I had been largely salon dependent and still I felt like my hair was spiraling out of control. I needed to figure out what was going on because these hair stylists didn't seem to have the answers. Armed with some key terms like damaged hair and protein treatment, I went to Google in search of instructions on how to take care of black hair. What I found was a treasure trove of information. I was reading all these terms and techniques that I had never heard before. I spent many nights and weekends reading about healthy hair practices and began developing a hair regimen for myself that incorporated hair treatments, clarifying my scalp, scalp massages, protective styles and so much more. Seven years later, I continue to use what I've learned to maintain healthier hair (and I'm still learning). My hair has never been this long or thick before and it's all been from the advice and guidance of the online healthy hair community. And like the circle of life, I share what I do with my hair to help others online who were like me.

References

1. Natural hair movement drives sales of styling products in US black haircare market | Mintel. com [Internet]. Mintel.com. 2015 [cited 8 March 2016]. http://www.mintel.com/press-centre/beauty-and-personal-care/natural-hair-movement-drives-sales-of-styling-products-in-us-black-haircare-market
2. Shah SK, Alexis AF. Central centrifugal cicatricial alopecia: retrospective chart review. J Cutan Med Surg. 2010;14(5):212–22.
3. Alexis AF, Sergay AB, Taylor SC. Common dermatologic disorders in skin of color: a comparative practice survey. Cutis. 2007;80(5):387–94.
4. Khumalo NP, Doe PT, Dawber PR, Ferguson DJP. What is normal black African hair? A light and scanning electron-microscopic study. J Am Acad Dermatol. 2000;43(5 Pt 1):814–20.

5. Quinn CR. Hair care practices. In: Paul KA, Taylor S, editors. Dermatology for skin of color. New York: McGraw-Hill; 2009.

6. Hair porosity types [Internet]. Naturallycurly.com. 2016 [cited 1 April 2016]. http://www.naturallycurly.com/texture-typing/hair-porosity.

7. How to Find the RIGHT Products for Your hair (Part 1: Porosity) [Internet]. Global Couture. 2014 [cited 9 April 2016]. http://www.globalcoutureblog.net/2014/07/determine-right-products-hair-part-1-porosity.html.

8. Kyei A, Bergfeld WF, Piliang M, Summers P. Medical and environmental risk factors for the development of central centrifugal cicatricial alopecia: a population study. Arch Dermatol. 2011;147(8):909–14.

9. Walton N, Carter E. Better than good hair. The curly girl guide to healthy, gorgeous natural hair. New York: Amistad; 2013.

Part IV

Hair and Scalp Disorders Secondary to Hair Care Practices

Seborrheic Dermatitis

9

Jean-Claire Powe Dillon, Cynthia O. Anyanwu,
and Katherine Omueti Ayoade

Introduction

Seborrheic dermatitis is a common and chronic inflammatory condition of the skin folds and areas rich in sebaceous glands such as the scalp, face, and central chest [1, 2]. Dandruff refers to scalp scaling without evidence of inflammation and has been shown to be a precursor to seborrheic dermatitis [1]. Though the prevalence of seborrheic dermatitis is thought to be between 1 and 5 % in the general adult population, some studies have reported a higher prevalence in blacks and Hispanics [3, 4].

Pathogenesis

The exact cause of seborrheic dermatitis is not completely known. It is often associated with overproduction of sebum, the oily secretion of the sebaceous glands [2]. However, this association has not been proven.

Malassezia furfur formerly called *Pityrosporum ovale* is a yeast that is naturally found on skin surfaces [5]. *M. furfur* may play a direct role in the development of seborrheic dermatitis and antidandruff shampoos are often directed toward eradicating this yeast [2]. *Malassezia* produces proteins that alter the components of sebum, forming compounds that cause inflammation in susceptible people [6]. Anti-inflammatory medications such as topical steroids are often used to combat this inflammation.

Stress, sleep deprivation, and seasonal variations in ultraviolet light exposure, humidity, and temperature changes have also been cited as exacerbating factors of seborrheic dermatitis [7, 8].

J.-C.P. Dillon, B.S. • C.O. Anyanwu, M.D. • K.O. Ayoade, M.D., Ph.D. (✉)
Department of Dermatology, University of Texas Southwestern Medical Center,
5323 Harry Hines Blvd, Dallas, TX, USA

© Springer International Publishing Switzerland 2017
C. Aguh, G.A. Okoye (eds.), *Fundamentals of Ethnic Hair*,
DOI 10.1007/978-3-319-45695-9_9

Clinical Presentation

Seborrheic dermatitis presents as hyperpigmented, hypopigmented, or erythematous plaques with greasy yellowish scales [9, 10] (Fig. 9.1a). It most commonly affects the scalp but may also be seen in other areas with rich sebaceous gland activity including the skin around the eyebrows, nose, and ears as well as the axillae, groin, and umbilicus. These lesions are often mistaken for "dry skin," especially on the face and ears, and are treated with over-the-counter emollients which often makes seborrheic dermatitis worse.

Severe seborrheic dermatitis is often associated with hair loss and occurs as a result of a variety of reasons. For example, because seborrheic dermatitis is often pruritic, vigorous scratching can cause a nonscarring alopecia (Fig. 9.2). Additionally very inflammatory disease can precipitate robust hair shedding called telogen effluvium. Patients should be discouraged from manually removing the scaly lesions on the scalp since this too can cause hair loss.

Treatment of Seborrheic Dermatitis

Treatment options for seborrheic dermatitis include topical antifungal, anti-inflammatory, and keratolytic agents [11].

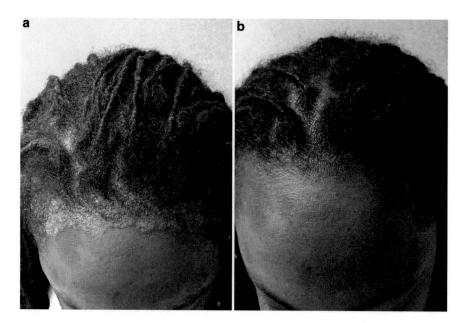

Fig. 9.1 (a) Seborrheic dermatitis in a male patient at presentation and (b) following 4 weeks of topical steroid treatment

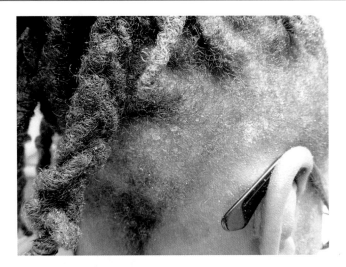

Fig. 9.2 Seborrheic dermatitis resulting in significant hair loss in involved areas

Shampoos

Ketoconazole 2% shampoo is a commonly used antifungal for the treatment of seborrheic dermatitis [12]. However, this shampoo can be very drying, particularly when applied to naturally curly hair. Ciclopirox shampoo is an alternative to ketoconazole shampoo and may be less drying. However, it requires more frequent applications to prevent flares [12].

There are several over-the-counter antifungal shampoos that can be used to manage seborrheic dermatitis. Zinc pyrithione, which is commonly found in over-the-counter antidandruff medications, is sometimes used alone or in combination with ketoconazole and ciclopirox to alleviate symptoms. Selenium sulfide, another popular over-the-counter medication, is also used for the prevention of *Malassezia* growth and also decreases the growth rate of cutaneous cells that contribute to dandruff and seborrheic dermatitis [12]. However, this shampoo, like ketoconazole, is also very drying. Additionally, it may cause residual odor and hair discoloration [1].

Keratolytic agents work by breaking down the outermost layer of the skin of the scalp, thus decreasing scaliness. Salicylic acid and coal tar-containing shampoos are the most common agents used in this class. Both can be effective at lifting excess scale, especially in those patients with severe disease. However, like many other dandruff treatments, these are known to dry out the hair. To combat this, patients may follow application of the shampoo with moisturizing conditioners and scalp oils.

For patients looking for a sulfate-free option, there are over-the-counter sulfate-free shampoos with salicylic acid, sulfur, and zinc pyrithione that may be good alternatives for patients with mild seborrheic dermatitis.

Topical Steroids

Topical steroids are commonly used to treat the inflammatory component of seborrheic dermatitis and can be quite effective (Fig. 9.1b). Steroids in oil or ointment preparations are generally a better choice for curly hair as opposed to alcohol-based solutions, which can dry out the hair. Although they contain alcohol, quick drying aerosolized foams may also be used, particularly in patients with chemically relaxed hair and others who prefer a lighter preparation.

Natural Remedies

Tea tree oil, derived from the leaves of the shrub *Melaleuca alternifolia*, has been used as an alternative treatment for dandruff [1, 12, 13]. This product has antifungal properties against *Malassezia*, and when used in a 5 % tea tree oil shampoo formulation, has been shown to decrease areas of involvement, improve itching and decrease greasiness [12, 13].

Additional Considerations

For patients with very curly hair, washing the hair daily is likely not feasible and this should be considered when developing a treatment plan. Instead, management should focus on increasing the frequency of shampooing to weekly if tolerated, and relying more heavily on medicated oils and ointments as the mainstay of treatment [14, 15]. When medicated shampoos are being used, patients should use a leave-in conditioner to moisturize the hair [16].

References

1. Del Rosso JQ. Adult seborrheic dermatitis: a status report on practical topical management. J Clin Aesthet Dermatol. 2011;4(5):32–8.
2. Bolognia JL, Jorizzi JL, Schaffer J. Dermatology Third Edition Volume 1. New York: Elsevier; 2012. pp 219–221.
3. Kenney Jr JA. Management of dermatoses peculiar to Negroes. Arch Dermatol. 1965;91:126–9.
4. Halder RM, Nootheti PK. Ethnic skin disorders overview. J Am Acad Dermatol. 2003;48(6 Suppl):S143–8.
5. Naldi L, Rebora A. Clinical practice. Seborrheic dermatitis. N Engl J Med. 2009;360(4):387–96.
6. Shi VY, Leo M, Hassoun L, Chahal DS, Maibach HI, Sivamani RK. Role of sebaceous glands in inflammatory dermatoses. J Am Acad Dermatol. 2015;73(5):856–63.
7. Emre S, Metin A, Demirseren DD, Akoglu G, Oztekin A, Neselioglu S, et al. The association of oxidative stress and disease activity in seborrheic dermatitis. Arch Dermatol Res. 2012;304(9):683–7.
8. Araya M, Kulthanan K, Jiamton S. Clinical characteristics and quality of life of seborrheic dermatitis patients in a tropical country. Indian J Dermatol. 2015;60(5):519.
9. McMichael AJ. A review of cutaneous disease in African-American patients. Dermatol Nurs. 1999;11(1):35–6. 41-7.

10. Sanchez MR. Cutaneous diseases in Latinos. Dermatol Clin. 2003;21(4):689–97.
11. Kastarinen H, Oksanen T, Okokon EO, Kiviniemi VV, Airola K, Jyrkka J, et al. Topical anti-inflammatory agents for seborrhoeic dermatitis of the face or scalp. Cochrane Database Syst Rev. 2014;5, CD009446.
12. Waldroup W, Scheinfeld N. Medicated shampoos for the treatment of seborrheic dermatitis. J Drugs Dermatol. 2008;7(7):699–703.
13. Satchell AC, Saurajen A, Bell C, Barnetson RS. Treatment of dandruff with 5% tea tree oil shampoo. J Am Acad Dermatol. 2002;47(6):852–5.
14. Silverberg NB. Scalp hyperkeratosis in children with skin of color: diagnostic and therapeutic considerations. Cutis. 2015;95(4):199–204. 7.
15. Lewallen R, Francis S, Fisher B, Richards J, Li J, Dawson T, et al. Hair care practices and structural evaluation of scalp and hair shaft parameters in African American and Caucasian women. J Cosmet Dermatol. 2015;14(3):216–23.
16. Hilton L. Caring for African-American hair. Dermatology Times. 2014

Scarring Alopecias Related to Hairstyling Practices

10

Alice He, Alessandra Haskin, and Ginette A. Okoye

Introduction

Over time, traumatic hairstyling practices can lead to both scarring and nonscarring forms of alopecia. In scarring alopecia, fibrous scar tissue replaces hair follicles, resulting in permanent hair loss. In nonscarring alopecias such as traction and chemically related alopecias, hair regrowth is possible but over time, repeated trauma can lead to permanent, scarring hair loss (see Chaps. 2 and 5). Additionally, hair styling practices can exacerbate existing alopecia. Understanding the role hair care practices play in the development of hair loss is critical to management of these conditions.

Central Centrifugal Cicatricial Alopecia

Scarring alopecias are disorders in which fibrous scar tissue replaces hair follicles, resulting in permanent hair loss. Central centrifugal cicatricial alopecia (CCCA) is a unique form of scarring alopecia that is characterized by a progressive, permanent hair loss that begins at the vertex of the scalp and spreads outward centrifugally in a relatively symmetrical pattern [1, 2]. CCCA is found primarily in adult black

A. He, BS
Johns Hopkins University School of Medicine, 733 N. Broadway,
Baltimore, MD 21205, USA

A. Haskin, BA
Howard University College of Medicine, 520 W St. NW, Washington, DC 20059, USA

G.A. Okoye, MD (✉)
Department of Dermatology, Johns Hopkins University School of Medicine,
5200 Eastern Avenue, Suite 2500, Baltimore, MD 21224, USA

© Springer International Publishing Switzerland 2017   111
C. Aguh, G.A. Okoye (eds.), *Fundamentals of Ethnic Hair*,
DOI 10.1007/978-3-319-45695-9_10

women with only a few reports in men or other races [1, 3, 4]. The average age at presentation has been reported to be 36 years [5, 6]. Prevalence data varies dramatically among population studies, from 1.9 % in a South African study to 59 % in a study done in the US [3, 7, 8].

Clinical Presentation of CCCA

Early stages of CCCA may present as hair breakage at the scalp vertex where short brittle hairs may be seen [2, 9, 10]. Erythema or follicular pustules may be also present in the early stages, although there are usually no obvious clinical signs of inflammation (Fig. 10.1a) [5, 6, 11]. Advanced stages present with a smooth and shiny scalp with occasional strands of hair (Fig. 10.1b) [5]. Associated symptoms may include scalp tenderness, pruritus, burning, and scaling [5, 10]. However, most patients do not have the aforementioned associated symptoms, causing the condition to progress unnoticed and often leads to patients presenting at advanced stages of disease [5]. Hairstylists can play an important role in early detection of this disease.

There is a grading scale for CCCA ranging from normal (0) to bald scalp (5) (Fig. 10.2) [12]. Imbedded in this grading scale are designations for the two predominant forms of CCCA: central (subtype A) and vertex (subtype B) patterns [12]. The central subtype is characterized by frontal accentuation, whereas the vertex subtype is characterized by prominence of the hair loss at the vertex. [12]

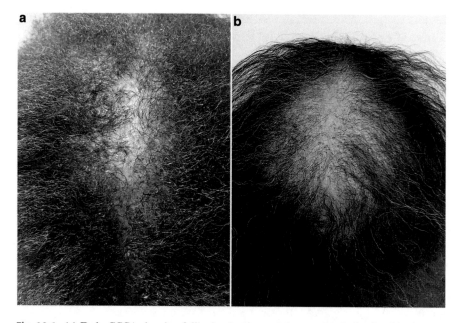

Fig. 10.1 (**a**) Early CCCA showing follicular dropout and decreased hair density (**b**) advanced stage CCCA

Fig. 10.2 Central scalp alopecia photographic scale in African American women (Reprinted Olsen EA, Callender V, Sperling L, et al. Central scalp alopecia photographic scale in African American women. *Dermatol Ther.* 2008;21(4):264-267, with permission from John Wiley and Sons.)

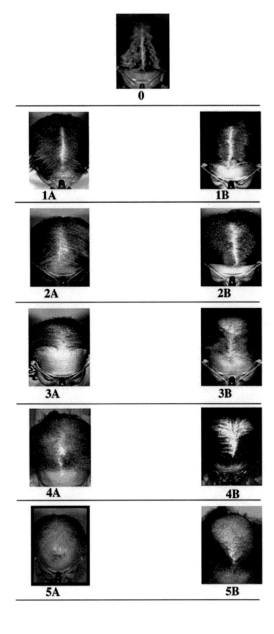

Etiology of CCCA

The etiology of CCCA is not completely understood but may be attributed to the unique hair grooming and styling practices of black women [13, 14]. As large epidemiologic studies have failed to demonstrate obvious associations, and other studies have found possible metabolic and genetic associations, the ultimate cause is likely multifactorial [13]. Hot comb use was historically thought to contribute to the development of CCCA, and the disorder was called "hot comb alopecia" until this theory was disproven. The disease was then renamed "follicular degeneration syndrome" since degeneration of the inner root sheath (IRS) of the hair follicle is an important histological finding in CCCA. The IRS acts as a seal for the nonkeratinized portion of the hair follicle [5, 15] (see Chap. 1). Upon IRS degeneration, this seal is broken. It has been proposed that bacteria and cosmetics commonly used in the hair care practices of black women (such as hair greases and oils) then gain access to reach the lower portions of the follicle, causing chronic inflammation and subsequent scarring [5, 15].

A number of interesting associations between CCCA and various metabolic pathways have been observed. In several US studies, CCCA patients were found to have a higher prevalence of androgen-related disorders such as hirsutism and acne, bacterial skin infections, and type 2 diabetes mellitus, suggesting that CCCA may be a marker of metabolic or endocrinologic dysfunction [3, 8, 16].

Defects in peroxisome proliferator-activated receptor-gamma (PPARγ), a transcription factor that plays a role in anti-inflammatory mechanisms and lipid metabolism in the pilosebaceous unit, are believed to play a role in some scarring alopecias [17, 18]. Defects in PPARγ have been shown to play a role in development of lichen planopilaris (LPP) and are thought to also be implicated in CCCA (see LPP: Proposed pathogenic pathways) [17].

Genetics may also play a contributing role in the development of CCCA. An autosomal dominant pattern of inheritance for CCCA was noted in a study of affected black South African families [1, 2]. In the US, studies have shown a family history of similar hair loss in the mother [5, 16] and maternal grandfather of patients with CCCA [8]. These findings suggest that there may be a genetic defect in the IRS in some families that predispose them to development of CCCA and/or shared family hair practices that contribute to development of the disease [5, 19].

Association Between Hair Styling and CCCA

More recently, development of CCCA has also been attributed to specific hair styling practices. Braided/plaited hair styles are quite popular among black women [5]. There are several different types of hairstyles that involve some type of hair braiding/plaiting, including cornrows, single braids with extensions, sewn-in weaves, and some types of dreadlocks (see Chaps. 4 and 5). These hairstyles have been associated with traction alopecia due to the tension applied at the roots and the extra weight that the additional extensions or long dreadlocks put on the hair follicles [5]. As these hairstyles are mostly unique to the black community and are associated with other hair/scalp disorders common in this population, there has been speculation that these same hairstyles might be related to the development of CCCA. Scarring hair loss and these traction-inducing hairstyles may also be related in a positive feedback cycle, as those hairstyles are more commonly used for camouflage in patients with the most severe alopecia [8]. It has also been proposed that CCCA may be a form of female pattern (androgenetic) alopecia that is exacerbated by these hair care practices [5, 20, 21].

Although two studies in the US found a positive correlation between traction-inducing hairstyles, such as braids and weaves, and CCCA, the largest multicenter epidemiologic study to date of central hair loss in African American women found no significant relationship between CCCA and relaxers, hot combs, or braided hairstyles [5, 8, 11, 16, 22]. Studies from South Africa also found no association between CCCA and relaxers or traction hairstyles [5, 22–24]. These data collectively suggest that the association between CCCA and hair styling/grooming practices in blacks is, at best, inconclusive.

Treatment of CCCA

Early intervention is key to prevent significant alopecia, as hair loss is permanent once scarring occurs [2]. The goal of treatment in CCCA is ultimately to stop further progression of the disease, rather than achieve complete regrowth of hair [17]. Additionally, the treatment plan should also focus on maintaining the health of the unaffected hair to improve the overall outcome. Unfortunately, treatment in patients with CCCA is often very difficult because patients seek treatment options at advanced stages when significant hair regrowth is unlikely and camouflaging hair loss is more difficult [6, 18].

Hairstyling Recommendations

Because specific hair styling and grooming techniques have been implicated in CCCA, it is recommended that patients avoid, or at least reduce, potentially damaging hair care practices, such as tight braids, twists, weaves, and cornrows [2]. Patients with CCCA should avoid heavy hair greases and hardening gels or sprays since they can increase the hair's fragility. They should also be encouraged to avoid using hot combs, flat irons, and blow dryers [2, 6, 10, 17]. In our experience, patients who adopt a "natural" hairstyle that is free of chemical dyes, texturizers, and relaxers tend to have better outcomes for two reasons. First, natural hair provides better camouflage of thinning areas as curly hair appears fuller than straight hair. Additionally, avoiding chemical treatments decreases the fragility of the hair that has not yet been affected by CCCA, and thus minimizes the chance of additional hair loss. Please see Chap. 8 for information about counseling patients through this transition.

Medical Therapies

There have been no randomized controlled clinical trials showing the effectiveness of medical therapies for the treatment of CCCA, but several treatments have been used with varying results [2]. Most of the currently available treatments are aimed at reducing inflammation [5]. Mid-to-high potency steroid ointments can be used to control local inflammation, while triamcinolone acetonide injections around the margins of the active areas can be used to prevent the spread of inflammation [2, 6]. These steroid ointments and injections should be applied at the peripheral areas of hair loss, including areas of normal-appearing scalp. The ointments should be applied 2–3 times per week and the injections done every 6–12 weeks [5, 25]. Antimalarials, tetracyclines, and other oral antibiotics may also help reduce hair follicle inflammation and bacterial burden [2, 6, 26]. Zinc pyrithione and ketoconazole shampoos may reduce pruritus and scaling [2, 10, 17]. Rarely used, mycophenolate mofetil or cyclosporine can help in recalcitrant active disease [10, 17, 27, 28].

Once the underlying inflammation is under control, topical minoxidil 2 or 5 % solution or 5 % foam can be added to stimulate hair growth on the scalp by extending the anagen phase of residual hair follicles [6, 28]. Hair transplantation is a treatment option that is only considered in patients who demonstrate an absence of scalp inflammation for at least one year in order to ensure that continued inflammation does not destroy the transplanted hair graft. [5, 10] A scalp biopsy is recommended to prove the absence of inflammation [10, 17]. Even without signs of inflammation, hair transplantation is challenging in CCCA because the presence of scarring decreases the hair graft's survival rate due to increased risk of infection and inadequate blood supply [3, 10, 17, 29, 30].

Lichen Planopilaris and Frontal Fibrosing Alopecia

Lichen planopilaris (LPP) and frontal fibrosing alopecia (FFA) are two related types of progressive scarring alopecia that share histological features. These disorders occur most frequently in postmenopausal Caucasian women but can occur in women of all racial groups including black women [31, 32]. The age of onset is usually between the ages of 30 and 60 years [33–35].

LPP is characterized by focal patches or diffuse areas of scarring alopecia on the vertex and parietal scalp, with associated symptoms of pruritus, burning, and pain in the affected areas when inflammation is present [33, 36]. Perifollicular scale and erythema are often present and are considered distinguishing characteristics of this disease [37].

FFA is considered a variant of LPP and is characterized by slowly progressive symmetric frontotemporal or frontoparietal hairline recession (Fig. 10.3a, b) [36, 38]. This band of frontal hairline recession may progress laterally to above and behind the ears [31]. There is often perifollicular erythema evident at the receding hairline, which may be a sign of active disease [31, 34, 39, 40]. Subtle hypopigmentation at the hairline may be appreciated (Fig. 10.4). Perifollicular scaling and hyperkeratosis are also common findings in the affected areas [31, 32, 41, 42]. Associated symptoms can include pruritus, pain, and burning of the scalp [31]. Although scalp alopecia is the predominant clinical finding in FFA, this condition has also been associated with loss of eyebrow hair and occasionally loss of body hair as well [31, 38, 39]. Bilateral eyebrow loss can be an early warning sign of impending FFA [31].·

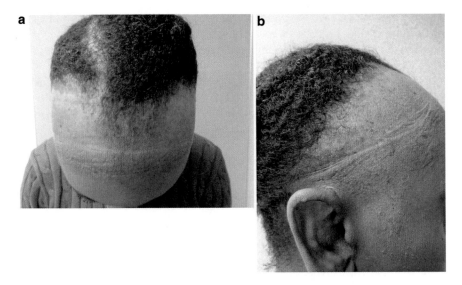

Fig. 10.3 (a, b) Advanced stage LPP. Posterior displacement of the hairline due to longstanding disease

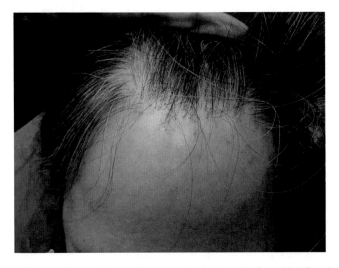

Fig. 10.4 Subtle hypopigmentation can be appreciated along the frontal hairline in this Asian patient with early stage LPP

Etiology of FFA and LPP

The etiology of LPP is likely multifactorial, with proposed genetic [40, 41], autoimmune, and hormonal factors. FFA has been reported in several families, although a specific genetic link has not been isolated [34]. An autoimmune etiology has been suggested, as FFA and LPP have been associated with relatively high prevalence to several autoimmune diseases, such as thyroid dysfunction and vitiligo [32, 35]. Some believe that LPP is an autoimmune disorder characterized by a cell-mediated immune reaction against keratinocytes in hair follicles [34].

Hormones are thought to contribute to the pathogenesis of LPP and FFA because estrogen affects hair cycle regulation [34, 38]. A study on the largest series of FFA patients to date found an increased incidence of early menopause in FFA patients, suggesting that low estrogen levels may be of significance [43]. The decrease in estrogen after menopause could alter the hair growth cycle and in some way trigger the development of FFA [32]. This would explain why majority of FFA cases present in postmenopausal women. The hormonal imbalance theory would also explain the reported effectiveness of antiandrogenic drugs (i.e., finasteride, dutasteride) in improving disease signs and symptoms. [32]

Treatment of LPP and FFA

There is currently no established treatment protocol for FFA or LPP and no randomized controlled trials have been performed, but several treatments have been reported with varying degrees of success [34, 38]. The therapeutic options for FFA and LPP include topical and intralesional corticosteroids, and systemic medications such as hydroxychloroquine, finasteride, and tetracycline antibiotics for more recalcitrant disease [33, 40, 42].

Conclusion

For all types of scarring alopecia, it is exceedingly important to educate patients on realistic expectations of therapy. Treatment may stop progression of the disease and relieve any associated symptoms, such as scalp tenderness, itch, or burning [5, 10]. Patients should be counseled that hair regrowth is not an expected outcome. However, in some patients, treating the scalp inflammation and addressing potentially harmful hair grooming and styling habits can result in improvement of the hair and scalp adjacent to the area of scarring alopecia. This results in improved coverage of the scarred area and can be quite encouraging to both patient and provider. As patients often find it difficult to appreciate small changes in affected areas, serial photographs are recommended in order to objectively assess improvement or disease progression.

Scarring alopecia significantly affects patients' self-esteem and overall quality of life [44]. As providers, it is vitally important to address the psychological impact of hair loss. Taking time to solicit questions from patients (and family members if applicable), addressing their questions and concerns about their diagnosis and treatment plan, and providing compassionate but realistic information about their chances for improvement engenders trust, and can significantly improve patients' ability to cope with their hair loss (Table 10.1).

Table 10.1 Coping mechanisms for patients with scarring alopecia

Providers can help patients cope with their diagnosis by:
- Ensuring patients thoroughly understand the meaning of scarring alopecia, the permanence of the hair loss, and the possibility that the hair loss may progress despite treatment
- Discussing the expectations of the therapeutic process. Patients can expect improvement in pruritus, tenderness, and other symptoms but should not expect regrowth within scarred areas
- Emphasizing to every patient that the primary goal is to prevent the progression of hair loss
- Addressing concerns about the etiology of scarring alopecia. Many patients believe factors such as diet, medications, and stress have caused or are contributing to their scarring alopecia
- Addressing feelings of guilt so that patients do not blame on themselves for their scarring alopecia
- Encouraging patients to include their significant others in the discussion and management of scarring alopecia, since they can be a major source of support for these patients
- Encouraging patients to include their hairstylist in the management process. Providers can communicate with stylists directly or indirectly by providing handouts with information about the patient's diagnosis and general care/styling recommendations
- Discussing camouflage options for hair loss and providing practical advice and resources
- Inquiring about patients' experiences with the therapeutic regimen so that necessary changes/compromises can be made to facilitate better adherence

References

1. Dlova NC, Jordaan FH, Sarig O, Sprecher E. Autosomal dominant inheritance of central centrifugal cicatricial alopecia in black South Africans. J Am Acad Dermatol. 2014;70(4):679–682.e671.
2. Madu P, Kundu RV. Follicular and scarring disorders in skin of color: presentation and management. Am J Clin Dermatol. 2014;15(4):307–21.
3. Callender VD, Lawson CN, Onwudiwe OC. Hair transplantation in the surgical treatment of central centrifugal cicatricial alopecia. Dermatol Surg. 2014;40(10):1125–31.
4. Khumalo NP. Grooming and central centrifugal cicatricial alopecia. J Am Acad Dermatol. 2010;62:507–8.
5. Ogunleye TA, McMichael A, Olsen EA. Central centrifugal cicatricial alopecia: what has been achieved, current clues for future research. Dermatol Clin. 2014;32(2):173–81.
6. Whiting DA, Olsen EA. Central centrifugal cicatricial alopecia. Dermatol Ther. 2008;21(4):268–78.
7. Khumalo NP, Jessop S, Gumedze F, Ehrlich R. Hairdressing and the prevalence of scalp disease in African adults. Br J Dermatol. 2007;157(5):981–8.
8. Kyei A, Bergfeld WF, Piliang M, Summers P. Medical and environmental risk factors for the development of central centrifugal cicatricial alopecia: a population study. Arch Dermatol. 2011;147(8):909–14.
9. Callender VD, Wright DR, Davis EC, Sperling LC. Hair breakage as a presenting sign of early or occult central centrifugal cicatricial alopecia: clinicopathologic findings in 9 patients. Arch Dermatol. 2012;148(9):1047–52.
10. Callender VD, McMichael AJ, Cohen GF. Medical and surgical therapies for alopecias in black women. Dermatol Ther. 2004;17(2):164–76.
11. Gathers RC, Jankowski M, Eide M, Lim HW. Hair grooming practices and central centrifugal cicatricial alopecia. J Am Acad Dermatol. 2009;60(4):574–8.

12. Olsen EA, Callender V, Sperling L, et al. Central scalp alopecia photographic scale in African American women. Dermatol Ther. 2008;21(4):264–7.
13. Miteva M, Tosti A. Pathologic diagnosis of central centrifugal cicatricial alopecia on horizontal sections. Am J Dermatopathol. 2014;36(11):859–64; quiz 865–57.
14. LoPresti P, Papa CM, Kligman AM. Hot comb alopecia. Arch Dermatol. 1968;98(3):234–8.
15. Sperling LC, Hussey S, Sorrells T, Wang JA, Darling T. Cytokeratin 75 expression in central, centrifugal, cicatricial alopecia—new observations in normal and diseased hair follicles. J Cutan Pathol. 2010;37(2):243–8.
16. Olsen EA, Callender V, McMichael A, et al. Central hair loss in African American women: incidence and potential risk factors. J Am Acad Dermatol. 2011;64(2):245–52.
17. Summers P, Kyei A, Bergfeld W. Central centrifugal cicatricial alopecia—an approach to diagnosis and management. Int J Dermatol. 2011;50(12):1457–64.
18. Karnik P, Tekeste Z, McCormick TS, et al. Hair follicle stem cell-specific PPARgamma deletion causes scarring alopecia. J Invest Dermatol. 2009;129(5):1243–57.
19. Dlova NC, Forder M. Central centrifugal cicatricial alopecia: possible familial aetiology in two African families from South Africa. Int J Dermatol. 2012;51 Suppl 1:17–20, 20–3.
20. Olsen E. Pattern hair loss. In: Olsen E, editor. Disorders of hair growth: diagnosis and treatment. New York: McGraw-Hill; 2003. p. 326.
21. Olsen EA. Female pattern hair loss and its relationship to permanent/cicatricial alopecia: a new perspective. J Investig Dermatol Symp Proc. 2005;10(3):217–21.
22. Miteva M, Tosti A. Dermatoscopic features of central centrifugal cicatricial alopecia. J Am Acad Dermatol. 2014;71(3):443–9.
23. Khumalo NP, Gumedze F. Traction: risk factor or coincidence in central centrifugal cicatricial alopecia? Br J Dermatol. 2012;167(5):1191–3.
24. Khumalo NP, Jessop S, Gumedze F, Ehrlich R. Hairdressing is associated with scalp disease in African schoolchildren. Br J Dermatol. 2007;157(1):106–10.
25. Hair diseases: medical, surgical, and cosmetic treatments. New York: Informa; 2008.
26. McMichael A. Scalp and hair disorders in African American patients: a primer of disorders and treatments. J Cosmet Dermatol. 2003;16:37–41.
27. Gathers RC, Lim HW. Central centrifugal cicatricial alopecia: past, present, and future. J Am Acad Dermatol. 2009;60(4):660–8.
28. Fu JM, Price VH. Approach to hair loss in women of color. Semin Cutan Med Surg. 2009;28(2):109–14.
29. Sperling LC. Hair density in African Americans. Arch Dermatol. 1999;135(6):656–8.
30. Rose P, Shapiro R. Transplanting into scar tissue and areas of cicatricial alopecia. In: Unger W, Shapiro R, editors. Hair transplantation. 4th ed. New York: Marcel Dekker; 2004.
31. Banka N, Mubki T, Bunagan MJ, McElwee K, Shapiro J. Frontal fibrosing alopecia: a retrospective clinical review of 62 patients with treatment outcome and long-term follow-up. Int J Dermatol. 2014;53(11):1324–30.
32. Vano-Galvan S, Molina-Ruiz AM, Serrano-Falcon C, et al. Frontal fibrosing alopecia: a multicenter review of 355 patients. J Am Acad Dermatol. 2014;70(4):670–8.
33. Lyakhovitsky A, Amichai B, Sizopoulou C, Barzilai A. A case series of 46 patients with lichen planopilaris: demographics, clinical evaluation, and treatment experience. J Dermatolog Treat. 2015;26(3):275–9.
34. Chieregato C, Zini A, Barba A, Magnanini M, Rosina P. Lichen planopilaris: report of 30 cases and review of the literature. Int J Dermatol. 2003;42(5):342–5.
35. Cevasco NC, Bergfeld WF, Remzi BK, de Knott HR. A case-series of 29 patients with lichen planopilaris: the Cleveland Clinic Foundation experience on evaluation, diagnosis, and treatment. J Am Acad Dermatol. 2007;57(1):47–53.
36. Racz E, Gho C, Moorman PW, Noordhoek Hegt V, Neumann HA. Treatment of frontal fibrosing alopecia and lichen planopilaris: a systematic review. J Eur Acad Dermatol Venereol. 2013;27(12):1461–70.
37. Meinhard J, Stroux A, Lunnemann L, Vogt A, Blume-Peytavi U. Lichen planopilaris: epidemiology and prevalence of subtypes—a retrospective analysis in 104 patients. J Dtsch Dermatol Ges. 2014;12(3):229–35. 229–36.

38. Chew AL, Bashir SJ, Wain EM, Fenton DA, Stefanato CM. Expanding the spectrum of frontal fibrosing alopecia: a unifying concept. J Am Acad Dermatol. 2010;63(4):653–60.
39. Armenores P, Shirato K, Reid C, Sidhu S. Frontal fibrosing alopecia associated with generalized hair loss. Australas J Dermatol. 2010;51(3):183–5.
40. Moreno-Ramirez D, Camacho MF. Frontal fibrosing alopecia: a survey in 16 patients. J Eur Acad Dermatol Venereol. 2005;19(6):700–5.
41. Navarro-Belmonte MR, Navarro-Lopez V, Ramirez-Bosca A, et al. Case series of familial frontal fibrosing alopecia and a review of the literature. J Cosmet Dermatol. 2015;14(1):64–9.
42. MacDonald A, Clark C, Holmes S. Frontal fibrosing alopecia: a review of 60 cases. J Am Acad Dermatol. 2012;67(5):955–61.
43. Martinez-Perez M, Churruca-Grijelmo M. Frontal fibrosing alopecia: an update on epidemiology and treatment. Actas Dermosifiliogr. 2015;106(9):757–8.
44. Haskin A, Aguh C, Okoye GA. Understanding patient experiences with scarring alopecia: a qualitative study with management implications. J Dermatolog Treat. 2016:1–3.

Pseudofolliculitis Barbae and Acne Keloidalis Nuchae

Chika Agi and Rawn E. Bosley

Pseudofolliculitis Barbae

Introduction

Pseudofolliculitis barbae, also known as razor bumps, is a common chronic inflammatory disorder involving the face and neck. Though classically involving the beard area in men who shave, pseudofolliculitis barbae may involve other shaved areas in men and women of various races.

Epidemiology

Pseudofolliculitis barbae (PFB) largely affects men of African descent with darkly pigmented skin and tightly curled hair but may occur in women as well (Fig. 11.1). This condition has been reported to occur in as many as 45-83% of black men [1]. Variance in the prevalence of PFB is affected by societal factors requiring a clean-shaven face in professional settings. PFB is less commonly seen in patients with fair or lightly pigmented skin and straight hair. Though not commonly seen in women, this disease may develop in the pubic area of women who shave or on the face of women with excess facial hair growth [1].

C. Agi, B.S.
University of Pittsburgh School of Medicine, M240 Scaife Hall, 3550 Terrace St, Pittsburgh, PA 15261, USA

R.E. Bosley, M.D. (✉)
Doctor's Approach Dermatology & Surgery, 2685 Jolly Rd., Okemos, MI 48864, USA

© Springer International Publishing Switzerland 2017
C. Aguh, G.A. Okoye (eds.), *Fundamentals of Ethnic Hair*,
DOI 10.1007/978-3-319-45695-9_11

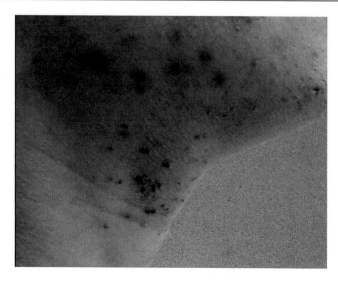

Fig. 11.1 Mild pseudofolliculitis barbae in a woman. Hyperpigmentation is common in ethnic skin and can take months to resolve

Social Considerations

The prevalence of PFB has risen with the increased popularity of multiblade razors and close-shave electric trimmers. Conformity to professional standards in various industries requiring a clean-shaven appearance has also contributed to the increase in pseudofolliculitis barbae. In the treatment of this condition, physicians must consider these societal factors and intervene when necessary to improve the patient's condition. For example, providing documentation to employers supporting the patient's need to avoid shaving can hasten the improvement of this disease.

Pathogenesis

PFB is thought to be caused by penetration of tightly curled, coarse hairs into the skin. The shaving of coarse hairs results in sharply pointed hairs which easily penetrate the skin, causing ingrown hairs and can occur in one of two ways. In intrafollicular PFB, the distal tip of the shaven hairs curls backward toward the skin surface and penetrates the surrounding skin 1–2 mm from the follicular opening. Transfollicular penetration occurs when the pointed hair is retracted beneath the follicular opening due to pulling of the skin taut during shaving. Once the tension of the skin is relaxed, the sharply pointed hairs pierce the skin through the sidewall of the follicle into the surrounding dermis (underneath the skin surface) (Fig. 11.2).

The penetration of the hair into the dermis induces a mixed inflammatory response. As the hair invaginates through the epidermis, a foreign body type reaction occurs. A dense mixed inflammatory cell reaction follows in order to encapsulate the foreign body. Subsequently, a microabscess and giant cell

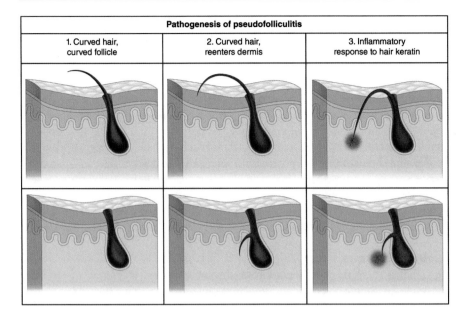

Pathogenesis of pseudofolliculitis		
1. Curved hair, curved follicle	2. Curved hair, reenters dermis	3. Inflammatory response to hair keratin

Fig. 11.2   Top row: Intrafollicular PFB—the distal end of the shaven hairs curls backward toward the skin surface and penetrates the surrounding skin 1–2 mm from the follicular opening. Bottom row: Transfollicular penetration—the pointed hair is retracted beneath the follicular opening due to pulling of the skin taut during shaving and pierces the skin beneath the surface

reaction occurs around the hair. Scarring may develop due to acute and chronic inflammation leading to fibrosis of the surrounding dermis [2].

Clinical Presentation

Pseudofolliculitis barbae classically presents as follicular and perifollicular erythematous papules and papulopustules in shaved areas. Commonly, this condition affects the beard and anterolateral neck. In severe cases, inflammatory papulopustules may evolve into abscesses. Chronic inflammation leads to fibrosis of the papules and eventual hyperpigmentation of the skin. Excessive fibrosis may lead to hypertrophic scar and keloid development. Chronic changes of the skin including rough, coarse texture, and scarring may occur in long-standing disease. These alterations in the skin can ultimately exacerbate the disease by making shaving and other hair removal techniques more difficult [2].

Approach to Shaving

Patient education is the most important aspect of the management of PFB. Patients should be counseled about the chronic nature of this disorder and the need for long-term treatment and adjustment in grooming regimens. It should be reiterated that the only way to cure this disease is to cease shaving the involved areas. For patients who cannot discontinue shaving practices, proper shaving techniques should be discussed.

Preshave Regimen

A careful approach to the shaving regimen is vital in preventing worsening of the disease. The hair-bearing facial skin should be prepared prior to shaving. Longer facial hairs should be trimmed to about 1–2 mm with an electric clipper or trimmer [1]. The skin should be cleansed with mild soap and warm water. The use of overly abrasive soaps or scrubs should be avoided. After rinsing the face, a warm towel or warm water should be applied to the face for several minutes. Additionally, entrapped or ingrown hairs should be gently dislodged with a bristle brush or coarse washcloth . A shaving cream or gel should then be liberally applied to the hair-bearing area.

Shaving Technique

The use of a sharp razor is important to prevent snagging or tugging of the hair (Fig. 11.3a, b). Single blade and multiblade razors provide varying degrees of closeness during shaving. Though multiblade razors may provide a closer shave, their use may cause the hairs to be cut below the level of the follicular orifice thus increasing risk of intrafollicular penetration upon regrowth [3]. While shaving, the skin should not be stretched or pulled taut. Hair should be shaved in the direction of hair growth using short, deliberate strokes. Overlapping of previously shaved areas should be avoided. Warm water should be used after each shave stroke to rinse out

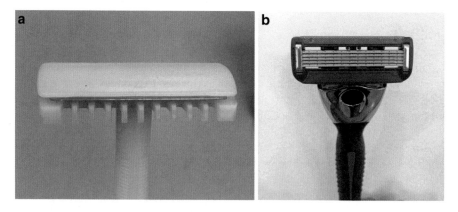

Fig. 11.3 (a) Single blade razor, (b) multiblade razor

hair that may build up between the blades [4]. The frequency of shaving has not been shown to affect PFB and can vary based on the patient's individual comfort and needs [3]. Once the shaving process is completed, the shaved area should again be rinsed with warm water. An emollient aftershave should be applied immediately. Aftershave products containing alcohol should be avoided to prevent unnecessary burning or irritation. In the event of pruritus or burning, a mild topical corticosteroid can be used to alleviate itching and inflammation. The use of mild keratolytic preparations containing hydroxy acids, such as salicylic acid or glycolic acid, can be used between shaves to soften the hair and prevent ingrown hairs [1].

Electrical Razors and Clippers

Electrical clippers are motorized razors containing comb-like blades (Fig. 11.4). Electrical razors or clippers are useful for controlling PFB and maintaining a hair length of 0.5–1.0 mm [5]. A hair length of 1.0 mm is achieved with clippers due to a protective gap between the blade and the comb thus preventing too close of a shave [4, 6]. Patients should be advised that unlike razors, which create a close shave, clippers may leave a stubble-like appearance that may be unsuitable to some men and most women [4, 6]. However, it is this feature that makes electrical clippers more advantageous than the use of a blade. If a closer shave is desired, clippers with foil guards or rotary shavers (Fig. 11.5) can be used as they have been shown to improve PFB [3].

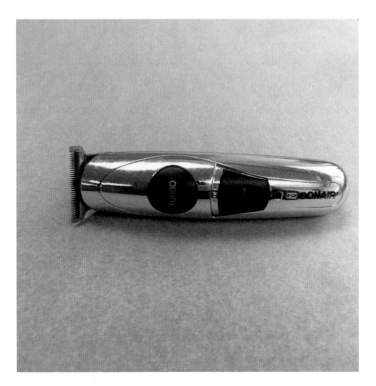

Fig. 11.4 Electric clippers

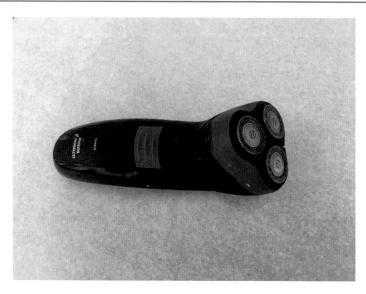

Fig. 11.5 A rotary shaver

Other Hair Removal Techniques

Chemical depilatories are used to remove hair in patients who prefer to avoid traditional shaving options. When tolerated, these products can be a very successful option for patients with pseudofolliculitis. Chemical depilatories typically contain barium sulfide, calcium thioglycolate, or potassium thioglycolate. These chemicals break the disulfide bonds in keratin thus weakening the hair allowing for easy removal. Depilatories are applied to the hair and left on for 5–15 min prior to gentle removal with a damp cloth. The duration of application is based upon the specific chemical composition [7]. Chemical depilatories are effective in dissolving entrapped hair preventing the inflammatory response. The chemicals only treat hair that has risen above the epidermis leaving all hairs below the surface intact with a blunt tip. The blunt end makes it more difficult for the hair follicle to penetrate the skin and cause ingrown hairs [4]. For this reason, use of depilatory creams can be useful in patients prone to PFB and are especially helpful for hair removal in the bikini area. However, these products are malodorous and can cause irritation of the skin. Using these products too frequently or leaving the products on the skin too long can lead to chemical burns. Lastly, effective treatment requires the hair to be grown to a visible length before removal can be achieved. This may be unacceptable to some patients, particularly women, and thus limits its use.

Treatment Recommendations Based on Severity

Mild Pseudofolliculitis Barbae
Based on the severity of disease, there are several approaches to treatment. Mild disease is characterized by both noninflammatory and inflammatory follicular and

perifollicular papules. The treatment of mild disease is focused on clearing the lesions so that shaving can continue. During the acute inflammatory phase patients will often complain of pruritus and pain. The use of topical antimicrobials and topical antibiotics (e.g., topical clindamycin and erythromycin) can decrease inflammation by reducing bacterial colonization within the lesion [4]. Benzoyl peroxide can be used alone or in combination with antibiotics after shaving. Patients should note that benzoyl peroxide has been known to bleach linens and clothing but does not have the same effect on the skin [5].

Moderate Pseudofolliculitis Barbae

Moderate disease is characterized by inflammatory papules, papulopustules, and fibrotic papules. In addition to topical antibiotics, topical retinoids and systemic antibiotics are helpful in controlling the progression of the disease. In mild to moderate disease, regular shaving can be continued while on treatment. Furthermore, alpha hydroxy acid products such as glycolic and lactic acids can be used to prevent hyperkeratosis and follicular plugging [1].

Hyperkeratosis plays a role in the pathogenesis of PFB, so retinoids are useful in reducing hyperkeratosis that often results from repeatedly nicking the follicular epithelium. Topical retinoids such as tretinoin and tazarotene, combined with hydroquinone, are recommended for nightly use to help improve clinical lesions of PFB and the associated postinflammatory hyperpigmentation [5].

Severe Pseudofolliculitis Barbae

In severe cases of pseudofolliculitis, strong consideration should be given to shaving cessation to allow inflammatory lesions to resolve. The hair may be trimmed during this period to a length no shorter than 3–5 mm in order to prevent further exacerbation of the condition. Topical antimicrobials should be used to prevent secondary infection of the inflamed lesions. Purulent lesions should be cultured. Empiric anti-*Staphylococcus* antibiotic therapy can be initiated while awaiting definitive culture results. For intractable disease, short courses of oral corticosteroids may be used to control severely inflamed lesions [2].

Laser Hair Removal for PFB

Laser hair removal is often an effective option in the treatment of pseudofolliculitis barbae (Fig. 11.6). Laser with wavelengths that target melanin is used to treat pigmented terminal hairs. Improper use of laser therapies can lead to epidermal injury and subsequent dyschromia and scarring, particularly in darker skin types. Long pulsed 1064 Nd:Yag and 810 nm super long-pulse diode lasers are commonly used to treat these patients. These wavelengths are generally safe and are less likely to cause epidermal injury. Treatment is given at 3- to 4-week intervals, often requiring four or more treatment sessions. Laser therapy can be used with topical eflornithine cream to accelerate hair removal. Eflornithine cream slows down hair growth by inhibiting ornithine decarboxylase. The use of topical eflornithine cream along with long-pulsed 1064-nm Nd:YAG laser hair removal has been proven to be more effective than

Fig. 11.6 Laser hair removal can be effective for the treatment of PFB

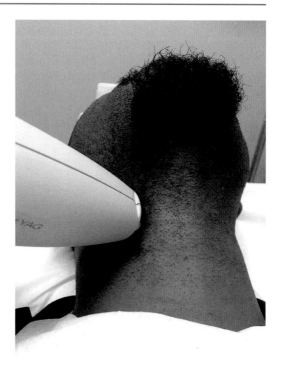

monotherapy with laser hair removal alone [8]. Hair removal with 755 nm alexandrite lasers and Intense Pulse Light has shown promise as a potential long-term solution for PFB treatment in select patients. However, the number of treatments required with these therapies may limit patient compliance. Effective treatment typically requires at least 8 sessions before improvement is seen [4, 9]. Intense pulse light is less effective in darker skin types and may not be a viable treatment option for black patients due to decreased efficacy and potential side effects [10]. Electrolysis is another option for long-term hair removal that works by using an electric current that is passed through a fine-gauge needle or flexible probe inserted into the skin, destroying the follicular isthmus and lower follicle [11]. Patients should be advised that electrolysis can be painful and often requires more treatments than laser therapy.

Acne Keloidalis Nuchae

Introduction

Acne keloidalis nuchae (AKN) is a chronic follicular and perifollicular disease characterized by firm, keloid-like papules and plaques on the occipital scalp and posterior neck (Fig. 11.7). Similar to PFB, this disease disproportionately affects men of African descent. Commonly, this disease has a chronic relapsing course and early intervention is vital in preventing disease progression.

Fig. 11.7 Acne Keloidalis Nuchae on the occipital scalp

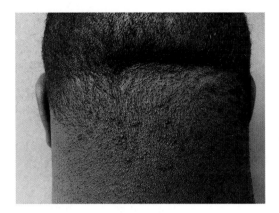

Epidemiology

AKN commonly presents in young black men but may also affect men of other ethnic groups. AKN can also affect women, though the prevalence is very low. Additionally, the incidence of AKN in prepubertal patients is rare [1].

Pathogenesis

The etiology of acne keloidalis is thought to be similar to that of PFB. Trimming or cutting coarse, tightly curled hair of the occipital scalp and posterior neck causes intrafollicular and transfollicular penetration of hair. There are many common exacerbating factors for this disease including wearing occlusive headgear or neckwear, including shirt collars. Patient may be prone to other follicular disease, such as PFB. A majority of patients with acne keloidalis may also have seborrheic dermatitis, which could be an inciting factor for a low-grade folliculitis [2].

Clinical Features

Acne keloidalis presents as itchy and/or painful dome-shaped follicular papules, nodules, and pustules on the posterior scalp and/or neck. As the disease progresses, the lesions evolve to more firm, keloid-like papules which may coalesce into plaques. Papules and plaques may present as discrete lesions or may form a coalescing linear distribution along the posterior scalp, which may extend to the vertex and parietal scalp. Advanced scarring and inflammatory disease may lead to alopecia. Additionally, tufted hairs and pili multigemini may develop near areas of scarring. Inflamed lesions may become secondarily infected leading to worsening pustular disease and eventual abscess and sinus tract formation. Though given the name acne keloidalis, early stage disease lacks the dense hyalinized collagen observed in keloid scars. Late stage scarring disease is marked by numerous plasma cells and actual keloid formation may occur [2].

Treatment

Early prevention is key to the management of AKN. Patients prone to AKN or who have early stage disease should avoid occlusive headwear to prevent irritation on the occipital scalp and posterior hairline. Avoidance of high neck collars is also recommended. There are indications that shaving-induced trauma may facilitate development of AKN. For this reason, use of razors or clippers should be avoided near the posterior hairline [12, 13].

Early intervention is important to impede the development of large, inflammatory lesions. The first-line treatment for AKN includes the use of topical antibiotics, topical corticosteroids, and keratolytics. For pustular lesions, topical clindamycin or erythromycin can be used with topical corticosteroids. Monotherapy with antibiotics can improve bacterial folliculitis and inflammation but may not improve papule size. Bacterial culture and sensitivity should be obtained for purulent lesions to tailor antibiotic therapy. Oral tetracycline class antibiotics are useful for extensive cases because of their anti-inflammatory and antimicrobial properties [5]. The use of high potency corticosteroids and topical retinoids can decrease inflammation and flatten papular lesions [2]. The use of high potency topical corticosteroids alone can improve mild to moderate cases of AKN. Topical therapies tend to be most effective at treating lesions that are 3 mm or smaller and are less effective at treating larger nodules. For larger papules and plaques intralesional injections of triamcinolone acetonide can be used to decrease inflammation and lesion size. Since AKN is a chronic condition, patients may be required to use prolonged treatment, which increases the risk of adverse effects. Patients are advised to take steroid-free treatment breaks to avoid side effects such as atrophy and dyschromia. In severe, recalcitrant and inflammatory AKN, oral isotretinoin therapy can be helpful.

Surgical Therapies

Surgical options for small, individual papules include punch excision followed by secondary intention healing or primary closure. The excision should be underneath the level of the hair follicle to ensure complete removal and decrease recurrence. Cryosurgery to individual lesions is also an effective treatment method. Best results are achieved when the lesions are treated for 30 s or greater though subsequent hypopigmentation may occur due to damage to melanocytes [2]. Laser hair removal is another option for the treatment of AKN. Long pulsed 1064 Nd:Yag and 810 nm super long-pulsed diode lasers are used to reduce hair growth on the posterior hairline to significantly reduce papule and plaque count [5].

The mainstay surgical treatment option for coalescing papules or small plaques is excision with primary closure. Electrosurgical excision with secondary intention healing has also been effective [14]. Perioperative treatment with imiquimod, intralesional triamcinolone, and/or superficial radiation can help prevent recurrence [2]. Radiation therapy has been used as monotherapy for recalcitrant AKN with favorable results [15]. Following surgical excision, the use of topical corticosteroids and antibiotics should be used to prevent further lesion development.

For large plaques measuring greater than 1.5 cm in vertical diameter, excision should be down to the deep subcutaneous tissue or fascia [2]. The excision should include the posterior hairline. Secondary intention healing is the preferred method of healing and primary closure should be avoided. Perioperative topical or intralesional corticosteroids should not be used as this can impede secondary intention healing [16].

Conclusion

PFB and AKN are chronic inflammatory conditions commonly affecting men of African descent. Due to intrinsic properties of the hair types in patients afflicted with these diseases, avoiding exacerbating factors can limit the progression of disease. Physicians must intervene during the early stages of these diseases as long-standing disease can be disfiguring. Patient education on preventative measures along with consistent treatment can assist patients in managing these chronic conditions.

References

1. Wilborn W. Disorders of hair growth in African Americans. In: Olsen E, editor. Disorders of hair growth diagnosis and treatment. New York: McGraw-Hill; 2003.
2. McMichael A, Curtis A, Gutman-Sanchez D, Kelly A. Folliculitis and other disorders. In: Bolognia J, Jorizzo JL, Schaffer JV, editors. Dermatology. Philadelphia: Elsevier Saunders; 2012.
3. Perry PK, Cook-Bolden FE, Rahman Z, Jones E, Taylor SC. Defining pseudofolliculitis barbae in 2001: a review of the literature and current trends. J Am Acad Dermatol. 2002;46:S113–9.
4. Daniel A, Gustafson CJ, Zupkosky PJ. Shave Frequency and regimen variation effects on the management of pseudofolliculitis barbae. J Drugs Dermatol. 2013;12(4):410–8.
5. Alexis A, Heath CR, Hadler RM. Folliculitis keloidalis nuchae and pseudofolliculitis barbae: are prevention and effective treatment within reach? Dermatol Clin. 2014;32(2):183–91.
6. Nguyen TA, Patel PS, Viola KV, Friedman AJ. Pseudofolliculitis barbae in women: a clinical perspective. Br J Dermatol. 2015;173:279–81.
7. Bridgeman-Shah S. The medical and surgical therapy of pseudofolliculitis barbae. Dermatol Ther. 2004;17:158–63.
8. Xia Y, Cho S, Howard RS. Topical eflornithine hydrochloride improves the effectiveness of standard laser hair removal for treating pseudofolliculitis barbae: a randomized, double-blinded, placebo- controlled trial. J Am Acad Dermatol. 2012;67(4):694–9.
9. Leheta TM. Comparative evaluation of long pulse alexandrite laser and intense pulse light systems for pseudofolliculitis barbae treatment. Indian J Dermatol. 2009;54(4):364–8.
10. Alexander AM. Evaluation of a foil-guarded shaver in the Management of pseudofolliculitis barbae. Cutis. 1981;27:534–42.
11. Shenenberger DW, Utecht LM. Removal of unwanted facial hair. Am Fam Physician. 2002;66(10):1907–11.
12. Kundu RV, Patterson S. Dermatologic conditions in skin of color: Part I. Special considerations for common skin disorders. Am Fam Physician. 2012;87(12):850–85.
13. Ogunbiyi A, Adedokun B. Perceived aetiological factors of folliculitis keloidalis nuchae (acne keloidalis) and treatment options among Nigerian men. Br J Dermatol. 2015;173:22–5.
14. Beckett N, Lawson C, Cohen G. Electrosurgical excision of acne keloidalis nuchae with secondary intention healing. J Clin Aesthet Dermatol. 2011;4(1):36–9.
15. Millán-Cayetano JF, Repiso-Jiménez JB, Del Boz J, de Troya-Martín M. Refractory acne keloidalis nuchae treated with radiotherapy. Australas J Dermatol. 2015. doi:10.1111/ajd.12380.
16. Bajaj V, et al. Surgical excision of acne keloidalis nuchae with secondary intention healing. Clin Exp Dermatol. 2008;33:53.

Part V
Special Cultural Considerations

Ethnic Hair Considerations for People of African, South Asian, Muslim, and Sikh origins

12

Crystal Aguh, Mamta Jhaveri, Alice He, Ginette A. Okoye, Brandon E. Cohen ,and Nada Elbuluk

African Hair Care Practices

By 2060, approximately 16.5 % of all US blacks will be comprised of immigrants, many of whom will originate from the African continent [1]. There were 1.6 million African immigrants living in the United States in 2012 and that number is expected to increase [2]. While more than 50 % of African immigrants are from one of five countries: Nigeria, Ethiopia, Egypt, Ghana, and Kenya, it is important to understand that the continent of Africa is comprised of thousands of cultures and ethnic groups, each with their own traditions [2]. Therefore, one cannot assume that the traditions of one country are also practiced in another. This chapter will focus mainly on cultural practices in Nigeria and South Africa, the sources of most dermatologic research on hair in the continent.

C. Aguh, M.D. (✉) • G.A. Okoye, M.D.
Department of Dermatology, Johns Hopkins University School of Medicine,
5200 Eastern Avenue, Suite 2500, Baltimore, MD 21224, USA

M. Jhaveri, M.D., M.S.
Department of Dermatology, Johns Hopkins University School of Medicine,
Baltimore, MD, USA

A. He, B.S.
Johns Hopkins University School of Medicine,
733 N. Broadway, Baltimore, MD 21205, USA

B.E. Cohen, BS
NYU School of Medicine, 550 1st Avenue, New York, NY, 10016, USA

N. Elbuluk, M.D.
Ronald O. Perelman Department of Dermatology, New York University,
240 E. 38th St., New York, NY 10016, USA

© Springer International Publishing Switzerland 2017
C. Aguh, G.A. Okoye (eds.), *Fundamentals of Ethnic Hair*,
DOI 10.1007/978-3-319-45695-9_12

Styling Considerations

Headscarves

Decorative headscarves are traditional head coverings commonly worn by women in Africa and the African diaspora. Headscarves can be made from many fabrics including brocade, cotton, or cotton blends and are individually tied to fit the head of the wearer. Referred to as "duku" (Malawi, Ghana), "dhuku" (Zimbabwe), "tukwi" (Botswana), or "gele" (Nigeria), these headscarves vary in appearance and functionality. For example, geles are colorful, elaborate headscarves worn by Nigerian women for important gatherings such as religious events, weddings, and dinners (Fig. 12.1). To ensure that geles do not unravel during the course of an event, they are often tied tightly and some women will even take a pain reliever before tying one for an event.

When worn infrequently, headscarves are unlikely to lead to any traumatic hair breakage. However, there have been reports of traction alopecia developing in women wearing tight fitting headscarves on a more regular basis [3]. When encountering an African patient with traction alopecia, dermatologists should enquire about more common causes of traction alopecia such as tight ponytails, extensions, and weaves. If the patient denies such hair practices, inquiring about the use of headscarves may help tease out the cause of hair loss if suspicion for traction alopecia remains high.

Plaiting/Braiding

Braiding is a common hairstyle popular among Africans of several cultural groups as well as people of the African diaspora. Braiding can range from simple cornrows to more intricately designed braided patterns and can serve as the primary form of hairstyling for many women [3]. Braiding the hair can be potentially beneficial as it allows the wearer to minimize trauma to the hair from routine grooming such as combing and washing the hair. For those who use braiding as a frequent styling option, they should be advised to avoid tight braiding, braid without extensions if possible, avoid chemical relaxers, and wear unbraided styles every few weeks to minimize the risk of traction alopecia [4, 5]

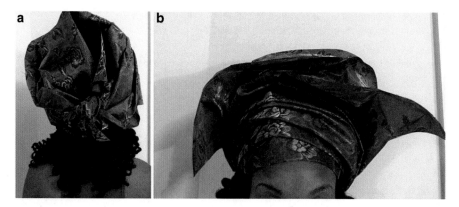

Fig. 12.1 Young woman wearing a gele

Chemical Relaxers and Extensions

Much of the research regarding hair and scalp diseases related to chemical relaxer use in the African population has been done in South Africa and Nigeria. As in the United States, use of relaxers and extensions is quite popular across the African continent. For instance, in South Africa, nearly two-thirds of women use relaxers to help straighten their hair and improve manageability. This proportion is likely similar in other parts of sub-Saharan Africa [6]. As a result, one will encounter many of the same adverse effects to the hair and scalp in these patients as would be encountered in the United States (see Chap. 2) [6, 7]. In South Africa, 17 % of schoolgirls and more than 32 % of adult women were noted to have traction alopecia in two separate studies [8]. Additionally, almost one-third of women reported hair breakage following chemical relaxer treatments in Nigeria [7].

It should be noted, however, that in most Nigerian public schools, girls are required to wear their hair chemical free and in short styles that are identical to those worn by boys [9]. For this reason, the use of relaxers, weaves, and other extensions is only permissible following graduation from high school. As a result, many see the use of relaxers and weaves as a rite of passage into adulthood. Continued abstinence from such practices may be difficult for those who have waited in eager anticipation for several years to use them. When encountering a patient from this area, this should be taken into account and dermatologists should encourage healthy hair care practices such as frequent conditioner use, moisturizing, and use of protective styles in those patients who are unwilling to discontinue use of relaxers and extensions.

Use of Plants for Hair Care

Like many cultures around the world, in many West African countries local plant products have proven effective over centuries to be beneficial for the skin and hair. Over time, these products have made their way abroad and are used by many ethnic groups for their cosmetic properties. Following is a brief discussion of some of the products dermatologists may encounter from their African patients and those from the African diaspora.

African Black Soap

Black soap, which originated in West Africa, has become a popular skin and hair product in the American market and other parts of the world. African black soap can be used to cleanse the skin or hair (Fig. 12.2). The exact makeup of black soap varies depending on its origin. It can be made from the ash of indigenous plants such as dried palm kernels or dried and roasted cocoa pods [3]. The Yoruba people of southwestern Nigeria are the originators of black soap termed "ose-dudu," which literally translates to "black soap." The most popular form of black soap is a combination of ose-dudu and the leaves of the camwood tree (also called "osun"). Together this forms "dudu-osun," which has exfoliative properties due to the rough texture of ground camwood [3].

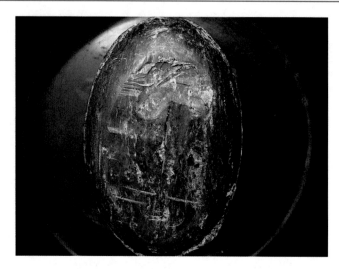

Fig. 12.2 African black soap is a popular product used to cleanse the skin and hair

Coconut Oil

Coconut oil is commonly used in Africa as well as other parts of the world for cosmetic purposes related to the hair [10]. As noted in earlier chapters, coconut oil helps retain moisture in the hair when used as a postwash agent and can impart softness to the hair [11]. Additionally, when used as a prewash agent, it minimizes hygral fatigue thus preventing damage and breakage [12]. Aside from its role as a hair product, the coconut has other medicinal purposes including the use coconut milk peripartum for relief of labor pains [10].

African Pear

Also known a Ube fruit to the Igbo tribe in southeastern Nigeria, the African pear is native to West Africa. This fruit is produced by the *Dacryodes edulis* tree, and in Nigeria the fruit of this tree are particularly large, with a thick fruit pulp [13]. This pulp can be used as a hair pomade but the leaves of this fruit are also used to treat nausea and wounds [10].

Velvet Tamarind

This fruit, native to West Africa, South Asia and Southeast Asia, is called Awin or Icheku fruit by the Yoruba and Igbo groups of Nigeria, respectively (Fig. 12.3). In addition to serving as a popular snack food, it is sought for its medicinal and cosmetic purposes. The powder of the velvet tamarind is believed to promote hair growth [10]. Other purported benefits include improving lactation and treating menstrual cramps.

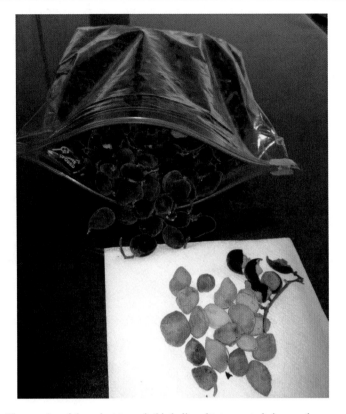

Fig. 12.3 The powder of the velvet tamarind is believed to promote hair growth

Cactus Pear

In the parts of the African diaspora such as the West Indies, the pulp of the cactus pear (*Opuntia* spp.) has been used as a hair conditioner and hair growth stimulant. The cactus (Fig. 12.4) is ground into a slimy semiliquid substance. It can then be applied to the hair after cleansing and rinsed out after several minutes. The pulp can be left in the hair to assist with freeform dreadlock formation.

South Asian Hair Practices

South Asian Americans are currently one of the fastest growing ethnic groups in the United States, representing approximately 1 % of the US population as of 2014 [14, 15]. The term South Asian American includes immigrants from the South Asian peninsula including India, Pakistan, Nepal, Bangladesh, and Sri Lanka. It also encompasses a wide range of religions, cultures, and languages. In this section, we will discuss a few cultural and genetic differences that will facilitate better understanding of the hair care practices of South Asian Americans.

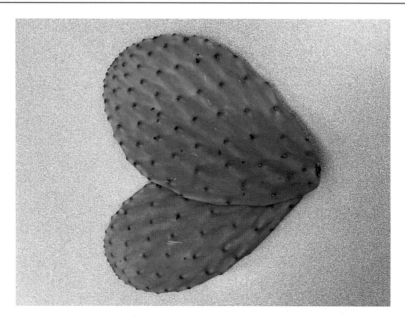

Fig. 12.4 Cactus pear. has been used as a hair conditioner and hair growth stimulant, and can facilitate formation of freeform dreadlocks

Hair Properties

To understand the cultural practices and products used to care for South Asian hair care, it is important to first understand South Asian hair. Although there are wide variations in hair type and genetics, the hair cuticle of South Asians tends to be wider and thicker than Caucasian hair [16]. The hair cuticle of South Asians can consist of up to ten layers. The hair follicles also tend to be close together with steeper angles increasing the hair density. Additionally, there is a thicker medulla, which provides added elasticity [16]. One source suggests that a specific gene may be associated with thicker hair in some Asians [17]. Because of the width and thickness of the hair cuticle and medulla, South Asian hair tends to appear thick and dark but also requires added moisture to maintain strength, texture, and shine. Without proper moisture, the hair is prone to hair breakage and split ends.

South Asian hair cuticles also tend to have a round shape, which helps prevent friction and tangling enabling the hair to get longer before breakage. Additionally, South Asians can have an anagen phase lasting as long as nine years, compared to the average length of four to six years [18]. Due to the long hair cycle, they tend to have less daily hair shedding. The hair shape, hair cycle, and texture, enable South Asians to have long, thick dense hair.

South Asian customs and hair care products have been passed down through generations to help maintain healthy hair [19]. For generations, thick, long, dark flowing hair has been used a symbol of good health and a woman's sensuality. By maintaining proper nutrition and hair practices, women optimize the strength of their hair by preventing hair breakage, decreasing friction and tangles, and maintaining the integrity of the cuticle and medulla.

Hair Oils

Hair oils are commonly applied from the hair root to the tip after washing one's hair to provide hair strength and shine. Hair oils have been found to provide a protective film preventing penetration of harmful substances [19, 20]. Hair oils also prevent hair breakage by decreasing frizz and tangles [19, 20]. Commonly used hair oils include coconut oil and amla oil, also known as Indian gooseberry oil. Although there are many benefits to hair oil, they can lead to heavy, greasy hair if a thick layer is applied or if it is used on thinning hair. Hair oils can also lead to contact dermatitis and folliculitis.

Amla Oil (Indian Gooseberry)

Amla oil (*Phyllanthus emblica*) is commonly used in India as the tree is native to the subcontinent. Soaking the Amla fruit in mineral, sesame, or coconut oil for 3–5 days makes this hair oil. Although there is no strong scientific evidence supporting its benefits, Amla oil is thought to have antifungal and antibacterial properties in addition to moisturizing the hair cuticle. Amla is also ingested to lower glycemic load and can function as a cholesterol lowering agent [21, 22].

Natural and Ayurvedic Shampoos

Shikakai Shampoo

Shikakai (*Acacia concinna*) is a climbing shrub native to central and south India. The Hindi word Shikakai translates to "fruit for hair." The shampoo is made using dried fruit pods, leaves, or bark that are ground into a powder or infused into water (Fig. 12.5). It can be made at home or bought in the stores. The bark has a naturally low pH and has been found to contain high levels of saponins, which results in the foaming similar to conventional shampoos containing sulfates [23].

Reetha Shampoo

Reetha (*Sapindus mukorossi*) is a naturally occurring soapnut found in the temperate to tropical region of the subcontinent. The shampoo is made by removing the shell of nut and immersing it into water overnight. Reetha has natural saponins that help cleanse the hair [24]. It is often mixed with Shikakai to make a natural shampoo.

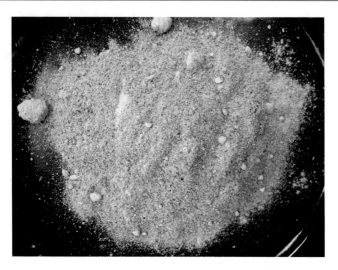

Fig. 12.5 Shikakai ayurvedic powder which can be used as a shampoo

Ayurvedic Shampoos

Ayurvedic medicine is a common traditional medicine system of the Indian subcontinent which is based on balancing the mind, bodily substances (*doshas*) and plant-based treatments. South Asians commonly use commercialized ayurvedic shampoos that are readily available which contain different mixture of herbs, including amla, shikakai, and reetha.

Hair Coloring

Henna (*Lawsonia inermis*) is a flowering plant that has been used for >6000 years to dye skin, hair, and fingernails. The dried leaf powder, which is green in color, is mixed with an acidic substance such as lemon juice, mustard oil, orange juice, or vinegar and allowed to stand. The paste is then applied to the hair for several hours before washing it out. Lawsone refers to the name of the orange-red dye that is characteristic of henna, and it permanently dyes the hair keratin (Fig. 12.6). The resulting color depends on the original hair color and quantity of henna used. If used to dye gray hair, the result is usually a reddish-brown. Henna can be mixed with other natural hair dyes including *Cassia obovata* for lighter shades of red or with indigo for darker shades of brown black. Many substances can also be added to red henna to enhance its darkening effect including tea leaves, coffee powder, charcoal, and turpentine. "Black" henna is usually a combination of red henna with p-phenylenediamine (PPD), which could result in a contact dermatitis in sensitized individuals [25].

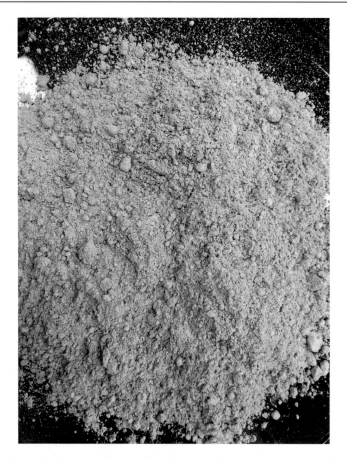

Fig. 12.6 Henna also known as "lawsone" can be used to dye and strengthen the hair

Eyebrow Threading

Threading is a popular form of hair removal in Asian countries such as India [26, 27]. In particular, it is popular among women for facial hair removal and eyebrow sculpting [26, 27]. There are several dermatological conditions that threading can cause, such as irritant dermatitis, folliculitis, bullous impetigo, molluscum contagiosum, vitiligo, and warts (verruca vulgaris) [26, 28]. Disruption of the epidermal–dermal junction during threading is thought to allow the human papillomavirus and other infectious dermatoses (i.e., bullous impetigo, molluscum contagiosum) to seed in the area of threading [26, 28, 29]. Threading also causes trauma that leads to erythema at the area of hair removal [26, 29]. Patients should avoid eyebrow threading if they notice any sort of rash around the face or eyes to avoid spreading infection or worsening a preexisting dermatitis.

Muslim Hair Practices

With a global population of 1.6 billion, Muslims comprise the second largest religious group in the world [30]. Islam is also the fastest growing religion, making it prudent for dermatologists to be aware of the unique skin, hair, and nail conditions that may affect this population [30]. Among these conditions, alopecia is one that may present with greater frequency among Muslim women who chose to observe the hijab [30, 31]. Hijab is the Arabic word used to describe the headscarf that is worn by many Muslim women [32]. It has many other names, depending on one's language and country of origin, but in general they all refer to the covering of the hair, which many women chose to do after puberty as an expression of modesty and to fulfill a religious duty. Muslim women must cover their hair in front of nonmale relatives, which means they are typically wearing the hijab in public but not at home or among family or other women [32].

Traction Alopecia in Muslim Women

One type of alopecia that may present in Muslim women who regularly observe the wearing of the hijab is traction alopecia [30, 31]. The hijab is typically worn directly onto the scalp and can be worn in various styles that can vary depending on the cultural dress of one's country of origin. Some styles involve pinning of the scarf under the chin, while others involve wrapping the cloth material into a turban or a bun at the back of the head. These styles can either be tight or loose over the underlying hair. In cases in which the scarf is worn tightly over the head, a continuous tension can occur typically over the frontal and sometimes occipital hairline [30]. This tension over time can lead to traction alopecia, which involves gradual hair loss and recession of the hairline. The location of the hair loss tends to correspond directly with where the headscarf touches the head. For many women this is the frontal hairline including the temples, also known as marginal traction alopecia [31]. For women who wear the headscarf as a turban or in a bun style, this can also involve the occipital scalp. Traction alopecia among Muslim women has been reported in the literature among several populations including Libyan and Indian women [31].

This traction alopecia is further exacerbated by the hairstyles worn underneath the scarf. Many women wear their hair pulled back either in a ponytail, bun, or braids. These hairstyles alone when worn chronically over time can lead to traction alopecia so for women who are also wearing tight head scarves over their hair, the issue becomes compounded and the hair loss is accelerated [31].

Prevention of Traction Alopecia in Muslim Women

For Muslim women experiencing this hair loss, there are several simple suggestions that can help. The first is discussing with the patient the way in which their hijab may be contributing to their hair loss. They should understand that in early stages this hair loss is reversible but if no changes are made, the continuous traction could lead to progressive and permanent hair loss [30, 31]. For women who are wearing it tightly, they can consider loosening the scarf in a way which still covers the hair but places less tension on the scalp [30, 31, 33]. Wearing their head scarf in alternative styles may also help decrease the tension which occurs from the scarf touching the same areas of the scalp each day. Furthermore, women can change the hairstyles they are wearing underneath their scarves so that they are wearing looser and varied hairstyles that also decrease the chronic tension being placed on the hair. Women should be advised that during time periods in which it is religiously permissible they should remove the scarf from the scalp and let their hair have a break from any tension [33]. Lastly, if necessary, these women can be provided the traditional treatments for early traction alopecia which can involve antibiotics, steroids, and minoxidil, as well as late alopecia which include surgical interventions and camouflage [31].

Hair Considerations in the Sikh Population

Sikhism is a religion followed mainly by inhabitants of the Punjab state in India [34]. Men and women who follow this religion make a lifelong commitment to avoid cutting their hair. Women suffering from hirsutism are not able to resort to hair removal practices employed by other sufferers of this disease. Dermatologists should be sensitive to this issue and should seek out aggressive preventative measures for Sikh women who are not comfortable with excess facial hair.

Sikh men are required to cover their hair with a turban (Fig. 12.7a, b) [34]. Before the turban is tied, the hair is pulled tightly in a knot that rests on the top

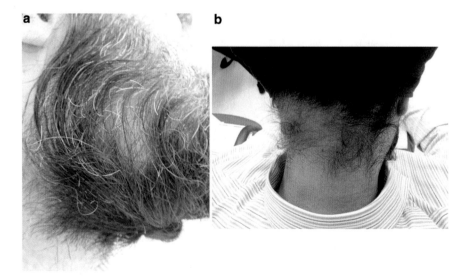

Fig. 12.7 Traction alopecia in the (**a**) beard and the (**b**) occipital scalp of a Sikh man as a result of chronic tension

of the scalp. This constant tension predisposes Sikh men to the development of traction alopecia. Similarly, beard hair cannot be cut and is instead tied in a knot under the chin. As a result, Sikh men may also develop traction alopecia on the submandibular area due to tying of their beard hair. To prevent worsening of traction alopecia, Sikh men should be encouraged to wear their hair loosely, without a turban, at night to allow for tension-free periods.

References

1. PewSocialTrends.http://www.pewresearch.org/fact-tank/2015/03/09/u-s-immigrant-population-projected-to-rise-even-as-share-falls-among-hispanics-asians/
2. US Census Data. http://www.census.gov/newsroom/press-releases/2014/cb14-184.html.
3. George AO, Ogunbiyi AO, Daramola OO. Cutaneous adornment in the Yoruba of south-western Nigeria—past and present. Int J Dermatol. 2006;45(1):23–7.
4. Haskin A, Aguh C. All hairstyles are not created equal: what the dermatologist needs to know about black hairstyling practices as related to traction alopecia. Journal of the American Academy of Dermatology. 2016;75(3):606–11.
5. Khumalo NP, Jessop S, Gumedze F, Ehrlich R. Determinants of marginal traction alopecia in African girls and women. J Am Acad Dermatol. 2008;59(3):432–8.
6. Khumalo NP, Stone J, Gumedze F, McGrath E, Ngwanya MR, de Berker D. 'Relaxers' damage hair: Evidence from amino acid analysis. J Am Acad Dermatol. 2010;62(3):402–8.
7. Olasode OA. Chemical hair relaxation and adverse outcomes among Negroid women in South West Nigeria. J Pak Assoc Dermatol. 2009;19:203–7.
8. Khumalo NP, Jessop S, Gumedze F, Ehrlich R. Hairdressing and the prevalence of scalp disease in African adults. British Journal of Dermatology. 2007;157(5):981–8.
9. Smith DJ. "These girls Today Na War-O": Premarital sexuality and modern identity in southeastern Nigeria. Africa Today. 2000;47(3):99–120.
10. Nwosu MO. Plant resources used by traditional women as herbal medicines and cosmetics in Southeast-Nigeria. Ärzt Naturh. 2000;41(11):760–7.
11. Ruetsch SB, Kamath YK, Rele AS, Mohile RB. Secondary ion mass spectrometric investigation of penetration of coconut and mineral oils into human hair fibers: Relevance to hair damage. J Cosmet Sci. 2001;52(3):169–84.
12. Rele AS, Mohile RB. Effect of mineral oil, sunflower oil, and coconut oil on prevention of hair damage. J Cosmet Sci. 2003;54(2):175–92.
13. Ajibesin KK. Dacryodes edulis (G. Don) HJ Lam: a review on its medicinal, phytochemical and economical properties. Res J Med Plant. 2011;5(1):32–41.
14. ACS Demographic and Housing Estimates – 2009-2014 American Community Survey 5-Year Estimate. Unites States Census Bureau. Retrieved March 1, 2016. http://factfinder.census.gov/faces/tableservices/jsf/pages/productview.xhtml?src=CF.
15. Pew Research Center Social trends for Indian Americans. [cited March 1, 2016] http://www.pewsocialtrends.org/asianamericans-graphics/indians/
16. Franbourg A, Hallegot P, Baltenneck F, Toutaina C, Leroy F. Current research on ethnic hair. J Am Acad Dermatol. 2003;48(6):S115–9.
17. Fujimoto A, Kimura R, Ohashi J, Omi K, Yuliwulandari R, Batubara L, et al. A scan for genetic determinants of human hair morphology: EDAR is associated with Asian hair thickness. Hum Mol Genet. 2008;17(6):835–43.
18. Kumar AR, Thilagavathy VR, Soleti P. Hirsutism: Indian scenario. Medicine Update. 2003;23:298–301.
19. Dias MF. Hair cosmetics: an overview. Int J Trichol. 2015;7(1):2.

20. Rele AS, Mohile RB. Effect of mineral oil, sunflower oil, and coconut oil on prevention of hair damage. J Cosmet Sci. 2002;54(2):175–92.
21. Mirunalini S, Krishnaveni M. Therapeutic potential of Phyllanthus emblica (amla): the ayurvedic wonder. J Basic Clin Physiol Pharmacol. 2010;21(1):93–105.
22. Amla oil for hair: benefits and uses. [Cited March 1, 2016]. http://www.enkivillage.com/amla-oil-for-hair-benefits-and-uses.html
23. Dubey S, Nema N, Nayak S. Preparation and evaluation of herbal shampoo powder. Anc Sci Life. 2004;24(1):38.
24. Upadhyay A, Singh DK. Pharmacological effects of Sapindus mukorossi. Rev Inst Med Trop Sao Paulo. 2012;54(5):273–80.
25. de Groot AC. Side-effects of henna and semi-permanent 'black henna'tattoos: a full review. Contact Dermatitis. 2013;69(1):1–25.
26. Lilly E, Kundu RV. Dermatoses secondary to Asian cultural practices. Int J Dermatol. 2012;51(4):372–9. quiz 379-382.
27. Abdel-Gawad MM, Abdel-Hamid IA, Wagner Jr RF. Khite: a non-Western technique for temporary hair removal. Int J Dermatol. 1997;36(3):217.
28. Verma SB. Eyebrow threading: a popular hair-removal procedure and its seldom-discussed complications. Clin Exp Dermatol. 2009;34(3):363–5.
29. Verma SB. Vitiligo koebnerized by eyebrow plucking by threading. J Cosmet Dermatol. 2002;1(4):214–5.
30. Desilver D. World's Muslim population more widespread than you might think. [Internet]: Pew Research Center; 2013 June 7 [cited 2016 March 15]. http://www.pewresearch.org/fact-tank/2013/06/07/worlds-muslim-population-more-widespread-than-you-might-think/
31. Malhotra YK, Kanwar AJ. Traction alopecia among Libyan women. Arch Dermatol. 1980;116(9):987.
32. Shah SK. Traction alopecia. In: Silverberg NB et al., editors. Pediatric Skin of Color. New York: Springer; 2015. p. 137–40.
33. Amer S. Arabs in America. [Internet]. Chapel Hill: UNC Center for Global Initiatives [cited 2016 March 2015]. http://arabsinamerica.unc.edu/identity/veiling/hijab/
34. James J, Saladi RN, Fox JL. Traction alopecia in Sikh male patients. J Am Board Fam Med. 2007;20(5):497–8.

Glossary

Acne Keloidalis Nuchae (AKN) Chronic follicular and perifollicular disease characterized by firm, keloid-like papules and plaques on the occipital scalp and posterior neck.

African Black Soap Originated in West Africa and can be used for the hair and skin. The most popular type, osun, is made from the leaves of *Pterocarpus osun* or *Okota osun* and acts as an exfoliator when applied to the skin.

African Pear Also known as "ube," this pulp can be used as a hair pomade.

Afro A natural hairstyle in which the hair is allowed to grow naturally, combed in an outward fashion, and molded into a circular shape on the head.

Aloe vera gel/juice Typically extracted from the inside of an aloe vera plant, is often used as an organic hair conditioner.

Amla oil Also known as Indian Gooseberry oil, this is thought to have antifungal and antibacterial properties in addition to moisturizing the hair cuticle.

Backcombing A method of locking the hair that involves teasing the strands to give a "ratted" look and then using a comb to push the hair towards the scalp.

Big Chop Refers to abruptly cutting off all chemically treated hair strands when transitioning to fully natural hair.

Bleaching Process that permanently lightens the shade of hair via oxidation of melanin. Involves the use of high concentration alkali solutions that can weaken the hair shaft leading to breakage.

Bonded Hair Extensions Type of hair extension that involves the use of bonding glue to fuse individual human or synthetic hair fibers to the base of natural hair shafts.

Box braids Hairstyle that is accomplished by interlocking three pieces of hair together in sections. Microbraids are very small braids, typically 2–3 mm in diameter.

Brazilian keratin straightening (Aka keratin straightening) a relatively new method of temporary hair straightening that involves the application of form-aldehyde-containing solutions followed by heat in the form of a flat iron to straighten the hair.

Carrier oils Also known as base oils or vegetable oils and help facilitate safe delivery of essential oil properties to the scalp and hair.

Central Centrifugal Cicatricial Alopecia (CCCA) A form of progressive scarring hair loss that most commonly affects black women.

© Springer International Publishing Switzerland 2017
C. Aguh, G.A. Okoye (eds.), *Fundamentals of Ethnic Hair*,
DOI 10.1007/978-3-319-45695-9

Chemical Relaxer Retouching Application of chemical relaxer to new hair growth only to avoid reapplication to previously treated hair.

Chemical Relaxing/Lanthionization Method of permanent hair straightening that involves irreversible cleavage of disulfide bonds within keratin molecules. Available in lye and no-lye formulations.

Co-wash The act of washing with a conditioner alone, instead of with a shampoo.

Coconut oil The most commonly used oils for ethnic hair care. This carrier oil has been shown to penetrate the hair shaft and is frequently used as a pre-shampoo treatment and moisturizing agent for both the skin and hair.

Cornrows Hairstyle that is accomplished by interlocking three pieces of hair that are laid flat along the scalp in stationary rows/lines or geometric designs.

Deep conditioner Thick cream conditioners that are formulated to be left on the hair for varying lengths of time (typically at least 10 min) to allow for prolonged contact with the hair shaft.

Dreadlocks Popularized by reggae icon Bob Marley, this hairstyle is created by allowing the hair to mat and knit together. Can be accomplished using several different techniques.

Essential oils Plant-based oils that are commonly used in hair care for their sensory effects on the scalp and their medicinal properties

Freeform locks Type of dreadlock hairstyle that is created by allowing the hair to knit together naturally into locks of varying sizes.

Fringe Sign The presence of thin, short hairs along the frontotemporal hairline. Characteristic finding of traction alopecia.

Frontal fibrosing alopecia (FFA) Type of scarring alopecia characterized by progressive symmetric hair loss along the frontotemporal or frontoparietal hairline. Considered a variant of LPP.

Hair butter Thick, semi-solid products that function as sealants which protect the hair against moisture loss.

Hair Tract or Track A type of hair weave that is created using machines that sew small pieces of hair together in a strip.

Head tie A traditional head covering commonly worn by women in western parts of Africa. Referred to as "duku" (Malawi, Ghana), "dhuku" (Zimbabwe), "tukwi" (Botswana), or "gele" (Nigeria).

Henna (Also known as Lawsone) one of the most commonly used natural permanent hair dyes. Colors the hair in shades of red depending on the duration of application.

Hijab A veil that covers the head and chest, typically worn by Muslim women.

Hot combing Method of thermal straightening that involves the use of a heated metal comb that is pulled through the hair.

Interlocking Quickest method to create locks. Involves the use of a latch pin (tool that hooks the lock and loops it through itself) or a crochet needle.

Lace Front Wig Consist of a thin piece of lace, extending from ear to ear, that is attached to the front of a wig. The lace is glued to the forehead.

Leave-in conditioner Conditioners that are designed to be applied following the use of shampoo and conditioner but are not meant to be rinsed out.

Lichen planopilaris (LPP) Type of scarring alopecia characterized by focal patches or diffuse areas of hair loss on the vertex and parietal scalp.

Lye Relaxers Chemical relaxers that contain sodium hydroxide as the primary active ingredient. Typically recommended for salon use only.

Monofilament Wig A type of wig that consists of a fine lace material in which hair fibers are individually tied to the lace.

Natural Hair A term used to describe chemical-free hair styling in people with naturally curly hair.

Natural Hairstyling The discontinuation of chemical and thermal processing techniques that alter the natural texture of the hair.

No-Lye Relaxers Chemical relaxers that contain guanidine or lithium hydroxide as the primary active ingredient. Can be formulated for at-home use.

Palm Rolling The most common technique used in hair locking. Sections of hair are rolled between the base of the palms. Can be used to start locks or re-twisting previous locks.

Paraphenylenediamines (PPDs) Primary component of synthetic permanent hair dyes. Can be a cause of allergic and irritant contact dermatitis.

Permanent Waving/Jheri Curl/S-curl Method of permanent hair straightening that "loosens" the natural curl pattern of the hair. Most formulations contain ammonium thioglycolate as the active ingredient.

Pineappling Pulling the hair up into a loose ponytail at the top of the head before bedtime to preserve one's hairstyle.

Pomade Solid emollient.

Pre-poo The act of applying an oil to the hair shaft prior to shampooing to minimize the risk of damage to the hair.

Protective Styling The use of hairstyles such as weaves, braids, and other extensions to minimize daily trauma to the hair.

Pseudofolliculitis barbae (PFB) (Aka razor/shave bumps) chronic inflammatory disorder commonly involving the face and neck characterized by curling of coarse hair back towards the skin surface resulting in erythematous papules and papulopustules in shaved areas.

Reetha A naturally occurring soapnut found in the temperate to tropical region of the subcontinent. The shampoo is made by removing the shell of nut and immersing it into water overnight and can be used to cleanse the hair.

Rinse-out conditioner Conditioners that are applied to the hair after shampooing and immediately rinsed-out with water.

Rod Setting Method of curling the hair that involves wrapping the hair around "rods" or "rollers."

Seborrheic Dermatitis (Aka dandruff) an inflammatory disorder that commonly affects sebaceous gland-rich regions such as the scalp, face, and torso. Typically presents with irritation, erythema, and scaling.

Shikakai Ayurvedic medicinal fruit that is often used as a shampoo.

Sisterlocks Type of dreadlock hairstyle that is created using a special looped pin tool. Referred to as "brotherlocks" when worn by men.

SLS (sodium lauryl sulfate) A type of anionic surfactant found in many commercial shampoos

Sulfate free Generally refers to shampoos that are free of anionic surfactants such as lauryl sulfates, laureth sulfates, sarcosines, and sulfosuccinates.

Tea tree oil From the leaves of *Melaleuca alternifolia*, a shrub-like tree native to Australia. It has been used as an alternative treatment for dandruff in patients

Thermal hair straightening Temporary method of hair straightening that involves the application of heat, which temporarily modifies.

Traction Alopecia (TA) A common, acquired form of hair loss related to prolonged or repeated tension on the hair root.

Trichonodosis Knots that form along a single hair strand.

Trichoptilosis Split ends

Trichothiodystrophy Genetic disorder characterized by fragile, brittle hair, and intellectual impairment.

Twist out A natural hairstyle that is accomplished by twisting pieces of damp hair around each other and "sealing" the hair by applying an oil or serum.

Twists Hairstyle that is accomplished by dividing small pieces of hair into two sections and wrapping them around each other. Can be held together using styling gel or beeswax.

Velvet tamarind A type of fruit native to West Africa that can be used for cosmetic purposes such as skincare and hair growth

Wefted Wig A type of wig that consists of a cap with machine-wefted rows of synthetic hair.

Index

© Springer International Publishing Switzerland 2017   155
C. Aguh, G.A. Okoye (eds.), *Fundamentals of Ethnic Hair*,
DOI 10.1007/978-3-319-45695-9